Ms. Cheryl McCray
144 Van Zandt Ave., Apt. 12
Newport, RI 02840

THE

†PRAYFIT ®

DIET

The Revolutionary, Faith-Based Plan to Balance Your Plate and Shed Weight

JIMMY PEÑA

and Eric Velazquez, with recipes by
Dana Angelo White, MS, RD, ATC

A TOUCHSTONE BOOK
PUBLISHED BY SIMON & SCHUSTER

NEW YORK   LONDON   TORONTO   SYDNEY   NEW DELHI

Touchstone
A Division of Simon & Schuster, Inc.
1230 Avenue of the Americas
New York, NY 10020

This publication contains the opinions and ideas of its author. It is sold with the understanding that the author and publisher are not engaged in rendering health services in the book. The reader should consult his or her own medical and health providers as appropriate before adopting any of the suggestions in this book or drawing inferences from it.

The author and publisher specifically disclaim all responsibility for any liability, loss or risk, personal or otherwise, which is incurred as a consequence, directly or indirectly, of the use and application of any of the contents of this book.

First Touchstone hardcover edition April 2014

TOUCHSTONE and colophon are
registered trademarks of Simon & Schuster, Inc.

For information about special discounts for bulk purchases,
please contact Simon & Schuster Special Sales at
1-866-506-1949 or business@simonandschuster.com.

The Simon & Schuster Speakers Bureau can bring authors to your live event. For more information or to book an event contact the Simon & Schuster Speakers Bureau at 1-866-248-3049 or visit our website at www.simonspeakers.com.

Interior design by Ruth Lee-Mui

Manufactured in the United States of America

10 9 8 7 6 5 4 3 2 1

Library of Congress Control Number: 2013036728

ISBN 978-1-4767-1472-1
ISBN 978-1-4767-1475-2 (ebook)

To Loretta:
My love, my life, my wife.
Any table feels empty without you.

Contents

PART III
The PrayFit Plan

PART I

FAITH AND FOOD: A POWERFUL COMBINATION

✝

Life is not about body fat and muscle tone.

It's about where our hearts are at and His grace alone.

It's not about the mirror or any other measurement,

but in our service to others, reflecting the Son He sent.

We're called to honor the body, but not for our praise or reward.

We're just simple, humble stewards, on a mission for the Lord.

So eat right, train hard, but don't forget your purpose,

God sees your heart and not what's on the surface.

1

OUR HEALTH IS
A MEANS OF PRAISE

Early Christians, in order to avoid persecution when they prayed in public, as well as to quietly identify themselves to other believers, would cross their fingers. Can you imagine if that was the only way you and I could share our faith? It's a subtle gesture, but it was a powerful one in those early days. In fact, by making that quiet sign, our predecessors risked their very lives.

What in your life says *believer*? If you couldn't say a word, what in your life would be that silent symbol, alerting another Jesus-follower that you are one of them?

It's a question I've been asking myself frequently over the course of the last few years, as I've been doing a lot of speaking to churches and to communities, as well as interviews on the radio, spreading the gospel of health and wellness. In the course of my outreach, probably the most common question I get from people across the country is: *Why are Christians known to be so unhealthy?*

And honestly, that question always makes me pause and wonder. Is that our silent symbol? Is *that* how we're identified by the rest of the world? Not by our love for one another, or even by our love of God, but instead by the way we risk our lives through neglect? My fingers are crossed that it's not.

Recently my wife and I visited a new church. We sang praises. We listened to a sermon about the importance of praise. Then, through tithes and offerings, we offered even more praise. All good. All expected. All right.

But then the pastor returned to the podium, patted his stomach, and jokingly bragged about the oversized meal and ball game he was about to enjoy. He even prayed that *it wouldn't be too healthy.* With my head bowed and eyes closed, I found myself squeezing my wife's hand.

You see, my life's work revolves around that fact that stewardship of our bodies—turning our heart toward our health—can be an act of worship. I don't believe that faith and fitness are incompatible. In fact, I believe that eating well and exercising regularly are actually directives from God Himself. It's an idea I've built the foundation of PrayFit.com upon, and I've spent the last seven years sharing our message with millions of people all around the world.

The truth is, eating well is not just a good idea because of the health benefits it brings, though those benefits are plentiful. I've seen firsthand how changing what you eat can change your life, whether you're a Hollywood actor (I've had the honor of serving as the exercise physiologist to Tyler Perry, LL Cool J, and Mario Lopez) or one of the countless church-going believers who have expressed to me the joy of finally establishing healthier eating habits. Yes, eating a balanced, delicious variety of foods will make you feel great (and will probably help you lose weight, if that's what you're after).

The real message, though, is that eating well is a good idea because honoring God with our bodies was His idea in the first place. At the end of the day, we're loved not because we've been successful at honoring Him with our bodies, nor because we plead forgiveness if we have failed at it—He loves us regardless— but shouldn't we be doing one or the other? The crux of my message is this: your health is a means of praise. It's a simple truth, but it bears repeating. *Life is not about the body, but our health is a means of praise.*

MORE THAN A MOTTO

Our health is a means of praise.

It's easy to say. It rolls off the tongue. But my motto is more than a line in a speech. It's more than a tweet or a Facebook status update. Of course, our body is only one part of our overall spiritual health. But as some of you have seen (and as I have certainly experienced firsthand), without our health, we just aren't going to be as effective in all the aspects of our lives that God needs us to be active in—our churches, our families, our jobs, our communities. Good health extends our ability to make an impact for the cause of Christ. Plainly said, God doesn't need our health to get His message around the world; we do.

Let me ask you something. What if nobody saw what you looked like? Would you work as hard as you do to keep your body in shape? Would you judge yourself as harshly when you looked in the mirror? Would you still watch what you ate, and would you make an effort to exercise? For some people, the answer is an easy yes. They have learned to love exercise for Heaven's sake, and they dig into a plate of healthy foods with delight and anticipation.

And then there are those who find making healthy choices a daily struggle. For many, eating well can be a challenge, because they equate indulgence, fulfillment, and satisfaction only with a plate of greasy, gooey decadence. But I'm going to show you a different way to approach eating and food. With the PrayFit Diet, you'll learn a flexible, creative way to put together delicious, filling meals that will nourish not only your body but also your spirit. And what's more, you'll find the resolve—and, even more than that, the *will* and the *desire*—to eat foods that will help you lose weight and gain health, because you'll finally see the connection between faith and food. Just remember that the by-products of your effort don't determine the worth of that effort. What determines the worth of our objective to eat better for ourselves, our spouses, kids, and friends is the One for whom we eat.

Friends, Jesus gives our lives meaning. He's the point of the story, the point of this book, and the point of our health we don't want to miss. He's *why*. For that reason alone, we place our trust in Him, and we pledge to Him our time, our money, our precious loved ones. And, yes, we should also pledge to Him our health, our commitment to living a healthy life—for His glory, not ours. The Bible reminds us that God sees only the heart. It also demands that we honor the body. That's not a contradiction. It's a priority list.

Taking care of the body through balanced eating is only *one* way to thank the Lord for seeing only our hearts. Every believer has been called to fulfill his or her purpose, but not one purpose calls for a neglect of health; not one. But if possible, forget the idea that when we're healthy, we're better at work. Try to ignore the fact that when we take care of ourselves, we're better for our families. Block all that out for a second. Focus on this short and simple command: *Honor God with your body.* Vain, you say? Petty? Too temporary? It *would* be if it were my idea. But it isn't. It's His. Once we realize that honoring the body is God's will, the result should be an unwavering, lifelong commitment to achieving that goal. But how to do that has proven to be problematic for so many of us.

HEALTH CAN BE A FAITH BATTLE

Now, when I say problematic, I'm speaking from experience, because over the last few years my health has been a faith battle. In fact, a couple of years ago, I wrote this in my journal:

> I never predicted such weeks like this. If I ever get up . . . if I ever hope and rise and stand . . . if I ever smile, truly smile and speak and write and encourage, make no mistake, it won't be because I kept fighting. It won't be because of my inner man, my deep faith or some gut-summoned passion of belief. No, I have none of that. If I ever get better, it will only be by the mercy and unbelievable, inconceivable grace of my dear God.

Indeed. See, while traveling, writing, and speaking, I was hit with two debilitating infirmities: one of the spine and the other of the colon. I came home to begin medical treatment, and over the next three years I lost fifty pounds of healthy tissue—not the good kind of weight loss. To help put it in perspective, I weighed more at age fourteen than I did at forty.

For years I tried to scale the walls of my pit, hand over hand. I was the perfect patient with an impeccable health ethic. But like many of you, I let go of the rope to find myself on my back, looking up at the impossible, knowing that God's grace is the only answer. I tell you, of all the things our health exposes, our frailty is one of them; a show of hands of those who can agree.

How many of you reading this today are dealing with unforeseen health issues that you're struggling to overcome? And how many of you are dealing with preventable issues? Whoever you are and whatever your needs, are you ready to conquer them? Well, trust me when I tell you that I know you can. How do I know? Because no matter what you're facing, He stops in His tracks for us when we call.

A few hours before my third surgery in three years, my wife, Loretta, and I were reading together about the blind man sitting on the side of the road in Jericho. His name was Bartimaeus. When Bartimaeus heard it was Jesus who was walking by, he began to shout out, "Jesus, Son of David, have mercy on me!" Over and over he yelled. Despite being rebuked by others, he continued to shout, "Jesus, Son of David, have mercy on me!" And it's the reaction of Jesus that touched my heart that morning of the surgery. The Bible says that when Jesus heard him shouting, He stopped walking. Some Bible versions say that He "stood still," and other translations say He "stopped in His tracks."

Well, friends, although I'm not blind, I *was* begging. I didn't want the Lord to take another sweet step. Seconds before surgery, a nurse tried small talk, but I'm afraid she sounded more like the teacher in the Charlie Brown cartoons. They transferred me to the operating table, which, for all I knew, sat on the side of that old, dusty road in Jericho. When the doctor said he would see me in recovery, before the anesthesia did its work, I slowly turned my head to the side, and as tears streamed from my shut eyes, I stole a line from Bartimaeus and fell asleep.

But the fact that you're reading this book means that Jesus stopped in His tracks for me. He stood still to hear a prayer. You know, when Bartimaeus received his sight, the very first thing he did was follow Jesus along the road. I suppose he figured the best test of his new peepers was to focus on the One who had finally made them work. I planned on doing the very same thing. And helping you gain sight of your faith as it relates to food is my highest priority.

But first let me tell you that healthy eating is not about a set of rules or a magic list of ingredients. It's not a matter of timing, food combinations, or calories counted. The reason I know this is because this generation is the most educated, the most aware, and the most capable of living a healthy lifestyle than any that has ever walked the earth, and yet we're the least successful at it. In fact, the next time you're at your local bookstore, mosey on over to the health section. You can't miss it. Ironically, the largest section in the store is reserved for the overflow of books written to help the world get thin again.

Without pulling a book off the shelves just yet, saunter through the thousands of titles. Explore the countless fads and innumerable strategies intended to help you and your family shrink: how-to promises from A to Z. One thing is for sure: none of them will work until you and I answer the bigger question of *why*.

See, *why* is both the question and the answer to the world's biggest epidemic. And it's a question that you won't find asked or answered among any of those books, until now.

THE QUESTION IS THE ANSWER

Determining your motivation for healthier living should go beyond the measuring tape. While starting points and progress checks are excellent tools for initial weight loss, things to bookmark as you diligently pursue the how-to of fitness, they do little to reveal *why* you're trying to get in better shape to begin with.

Your personal *why* may be sitting across from you at the kitchen table. Those giggling kids need a healthy role model around. Or maybe you're sitting with your chin resting in your hand, looking at one of your parents—your mom moved in with you after your dad passed away, and not only does she have specific food-related needs, but you need the strength and stamina to care for a family and to care for the parent who raised you.

Your *why* may greet you in the mirror each morning. The years of neglect haven't been good to your lungs, your blood pressure, or your reflection. Knowing God looks at the heart is simultaneously comforting and convicting, since willful neglect can be a soul's inward reality with an outward brutality.

Your *why* may be the mere fact that you are fearfully and wonderfully made. You know that God spoke, and there was light. He breathed the stars into space and put the moon in place. But you? You, He knitted. Imagine that the God who filled the oceans with water made your eyes to blink. After spraying the cosmos with trillions of galaxies, He gave you goose bumps. (And then you did the same to Him.)

See, before your very first day of school, or prior to getting your driver's license, and even before you began the family with which you spend your days . . . came your body. Not only did God inspire your soul's dream but He gave you the body necessary to pursue the job. Since God will always equip us with what we need to accomplish His will, we know our bodies were *His* choice. Can you imagine the moment? It was as if God said: "Sweet soul, here is your body. I've carefully woven it together. It has what it takes for you to pursue Me and tell others about Me. Precious body, this is your soul. Of all the matter in the universe, this is what matters most. Carry it where it needs to go. Protect it. Honor it. Now, I want you two to be good to each other. Be friends, not enemies."

Humor me for a second and take a quick glance at your arm or hands. Think for a second that God Himself has *touched* that skin. He was first. In fact, talk to your body. It's okay, go ahead. Maybe you need to thank it. Perhaps you need to reassure it. Or maybe you need to apologize for not paying more attention to the foods you've been indulging in. But much as you would with any friend going through a tough time, just tell it you're so very sorry. After all, it was God who knitted it and then breathed life into it. Miraculously, He gave your heart knowledge that there is something more to this life than life. Your soul and your body are a match *made* in Heaven.

Because of that match, we are capable defenders. It's funny— we put locks on our doors at home and security systems in our cars, we spam-proof our e-mails and put passwords on our phones, we stand at the gates of the most important elements in life. But when it comes to food choices, we're much less protective. Although we're armed with knowledge, *that* guard is fast asleep outside our door. We've offered diabetes, heart disease, and obesity the keys to their favorite rooms as they check in.

But folks, we *are* capable defenders. Like it says in 1 Corinthians 9:17, we have been entrusted with stewardship. When God said to honor Him with our bodies, we became guardians of health. Our eternity is His responsibility; we can't earn it. Fortunately for us, He put us in charge of something that requires our effort. And when it comes to our health, it begins at the table.

THAT'S THE ONE

Now, at this point, I'm going to assume that if you're reading this page, you're still with me. You're not quite ready to shove this title back onto the shelf. I'm glad. I'm going to assume that you have a good idea of your own personal *why* factor and you're ready for battle. You just need to know where the fight is.

Reminds me of David. See, before young David hurled the stone at the giant, I picture him down at the stream, picking the stones up one at a time and weighing them in his hand. See, I have a feeling he measured a few before finding *just* the right one for his particular overgrown nuisance.

In 1 Samuel 17:40 the Bible says, "Then he took his staff in his hand, and chose five smooth stones from the stream." Did you notice the word used there? He *chose* five stones. He made *decisions* based on his needs and abilities. That one's too light—toss it. That one's too small—toss. Ah, *that's* the one! After all, David knew what he was up against and planned accordingly. Not only that, he chose five stones, not because he thought he would miss, but because David knew Goliath had brothers.

What about you? In the area of healthy eating, you or your loved ones might be facing some big issues: obesity and his brothers heart disease and diabetes. If so, it's time to take a stroll down to the stream with David. Kneel down with him and gather some ammo. If the pebbles you've been flinging at your giant-sized goals aren't making a dent, then it's time to reload. You know what you're up against. The key is to do like David did and find the right stone. Remember, his fight was worth it, and so is yours.

That's the purpose of this book. You've come to the stream, and the PrayFit Diet is exactly what you need to slay your giant. You've broken through the excuses and the muck of empty how-to information to say, "Enough is enough!" Because you've changed from the inside out, you're ready for your body weight, blood pressure, or dress size to be a by-product of obedience. You know your *why*; we are blessed to show you *how*.

PRAYFIT EATING 101

The PrayFit Diet is arguably the most balanced food plan ever assembled, harnessing the best elements of the food we were always meant to eat. Unlike other diets, which tell you to cut out a whole category of food so you will quickly shed pounds—only to gain it back (and then some) once you resume normal eating—PrayFit is a sustainable way of eating because it's a *balanced* way of eating. On PrayFit, you'll eat protein, fat, and carbs, all in equal caloric proportions. Perfect harmony. The better able you are to put these macronutrients to use each day, the quicker you'll lose weight, gain confidence, and begin a lifestyle of long-lasting, healthy change.

Nowhere in these pages will you find calls for radical depriva-tion, the elimination of entire food groups, or confounding and discouraging food measurements. On the contrary, you find bal-ance, abundance, simplicity, and sustainability. I'll get into more of the details of the PrayFit Diet as we get deeper into the book, but here's what you need to know now.

BALANCE. Calories matter, but it is the distribution of calories through food types that will play a crucial role in energy, me-tabolism, and body composition. The PrayFit Diet provides equal amounts of calories from healthy sources of protein, carbs, and fat—33 percent of your day's take from each—allowing you to capitalize on the body and brain benefits of each.

ABUNDANCE. As a nation, perhaps we can stand to eat a little less, but that is not the best long-term solution for a radical change in our health. The PrayFit Diet teaches the value of each of the macronutrients, instead of viewing them as competing food sources. Protein, carbs, and fat are all important to health, per-formance, and weight loss. We show you how to enjoy them all in abundance while continuing to see change in your body.

SIMPLICITY. If you've ever tried a dietary plan that calls for count-ing calories or measuring things down to the half ounce, you've no doubt dealt with the frustration that it can produce. By insist-ing on balance and illustrating practical ways of planning meals, we forgo these expected, complicated dietary hurdles and leave you with an eye—and heart—for easy, healthy eating.

SUSTAINABILITY. Our goal isn't just to help you lose weight this month. It's to help you reach your goal weight, no matter how long it takes, and then to help you maintain it for as long as your lungs have breath. The absence of extreme deprivation combined with the inclusion of health-boosting dietary balance makes the

PrayFit Diet a resource that you can come back to again and again for years to come. No monthlong "cycle off," no "coming back to it when you're ready"—this plan is designed to help you to rethink the way you view nutrition and to flourish physically, forever.

FAITH MATTERS

You know the feeling. I do, too. Bottom of the ninth, two outs, and your favorite batter hits one deep. You stand, your eyes widen, your mouth opens! It's going, going...*caught.* That's the ball game—your team loses. But for a few short seconds the thrill of what might be did a tap dance on your heart. And it felt great while it lasted. Really, really great.

You've probably experienced this momentary elation on other diets, too—an early excitement as you started to see the pounds fall away, only to have it followed by a crushing disappointment when you realized that the plan wasn't sustainable in the long term and you were right back where you'd started. This book gives you a thirty-three-day plan to get started on the PrayFit Diet. But this is not a short-term fix. It's a long-term, healthy way of eating, one that you can sustain for months and years to come.

You and I were designed to live abundant, active, healthy lives. If there's one thing we know, He designed and can repair what we mess up. From our hearts to our health problems, He cares. He really *cares.* And because He does, we have permission to pursue slimmer waistlines and lower blood pressure. In 3 John, the apostle writes to his readers, "I hope you are as healthy in body, as you are strong in spirit." See, John knew how important our bodies were to accomplishing and conquering this life. He understood that this body is God's house. He understood that our souls have work to do within our homes, communities, churches, and schools, and nothing—*nothing,* especially our bodies—should be holding us back.

What follows in these pages is a road map to a better, healthier body—a plan that is markedly divergent from the deluge of how-to diets that litter shelves, blogs, and infomercials from here to eternity. And eternity is the reason. The PrayFit Diet isn't just about the mechanics of healthier eating but about the motivations for faithful *living*. That our bodies happen to be intimately tied to our purpose on this earth is something that we may not always pause to take stock of. We'll help you to make the connection, putting you on a path to effective, faith-driven stewardship of your body. Those of you who commit fully to the program can lose twenty pounds in the next thirty-three days if that's your goal, but the lifestyle you'll create far outweighs the weight you'll lose—and what your body can *and will* achieve for God's purpose in your life is why.

In Part I of the book, I'll give you an overview of the PrayFit Diet and explain the foundation (both the health foundation and the biblical foundation) of this powerful new way of eating. In Part II, I'll take you through the three macronutrients that will make up your PrayFit Plate: protein, fat, and carbohydrates. And in Part III, we'll put it all into practice, with a five week guide to shopping, cooking, and eating the PrayFit way.

Read on, and learn how to make the PrayFit Diet work for you to feed your body, nourish your spirit, and support the kind of life you were always meant to live.

†

*O*ur *diligence toward a healthier lifestyle*
is not about the mirror. It's about the One
we're trying to mirror.

2

THE SIMPLE 33 BALANCE

HOW BALANCING PROTEIN, FAT, AND CARBS IS THE
KEY TO LOSING WEIGHT AND KEEPING IT OFF

I have a long list of goals. Wanna hear a few of them? Okay, here goes. In no particular order—and *before* I turn fifty—my goals are to (1) become fluent in Spanish, (2) memorize the New Testament, (3) learn to play the piano, (4) visit Bethlehem, and (5) be able to do a handstand.

Do you like my odds? (Please, no bets on the handstand.)

Do you see any common denominators to my life's objectives? I can think of two: God's will and my health. I am nothing without either. But I love to imagine all the things I could do with God's blessing of a plan *and* His blessing of good health to see it through. Wow. The idea literally makes my heart pound. Friends, I'm convinced that the only two elements any believer needs when it comes to his or her goals are God's will and health.

That balance puts us in a position to do incredible things, pursue dreams, and achieve real joy.

So how do we get to this balanced place of health? First off, I will say that there's a great deal that is under your control when it comes to making healthy choices. But as someone who has been on the front lines of the health industry for more than a decade, I'm here to tell you that there's a lot of misinformation out there, too. It's often really hard for people to sift through all the conflicting messages about food and fitness to understand what they need to do to get healthy. I want to help you cut through all the hype.

Somewhere along the way, *diet* became a catchword used to describe a temporary way of eating designed to get you to lose weight faster. Some diets deliver on their promises rather quickly, only to see you gain it all back—and then some—in a month or two. Unfortunately, the architects of these fad diets have become masters at making their product stand out in a crowded market without ever illuminating *why* you should be working toward weight loss in the first place. In the absence of clarity of purpose, a return to previous habits— and previous weight—is nearly inevitable.

What's more problematic is that these programs are often fraught with assurances of the weight loss that is to come, usually at the expense of genuine education. Four weeks of skimping on carbs and calories, as some of you may already know, is a maddeningly frustrating exercise that leaves the dieter dazed and lethargic—hardly the picture of abundant health, even if you are (temporarily) a few pounds lighter. Unless you are walking around with an advanced degree in nutrition, you're not likely to question the information presented to you.

Any nutrition plan based on deprivation is simply unsustainable. What's more, you don't learn anything from fad diets.

Once you're faced with all kinds of foods again, you gain back the weight you lost and sometimes more. Thankfully, God designed us to eat things in balance, hence the abundance of food sources made available to us from the beginning.

> Then God said, "I give you every seed-bearing plant on the face of the whole earth and every tree that has fruit with seed in it. They will be yours for food. And to all the beasts of the earth and all the birds of the air and all the creatures that move on the ground—everything that has the breath of life in it—I give every green plant for food." And it was so.
>
> (GENESIS 1:29–30)

And you have to keep in mind that a single dietary indiscretion does not lead to unhealthy weight or higher blood pressure. Usually a pattern emerges that leads to unintended consequences. We begin to eat beyond satiety. We begin to associate food with comfort. We begin to lose sight of food's true purpose— to provide the fuel we need to do the Lord's work. When we allow our concept of food to be corrupted by a society quick to overindulge, we can pay a steep price, both physically and spiritually. We need a change in heart.

Though it should be enjoyed, food isn't a reward so much as it is a blessing provided to you by a kind and loving God who cares for your health and well-being. To arbitrarily redefine food's purpose is to mock the provision of it and ignore its intended purpose.

> So whether you eat or drink or whatever you do, do it all for the glory of God.
>
> (I CORINTHIANS 10:31)

WHAT IS BALANCE?

Some programs will try to sell you on the idea that all calories are created equal, but that is simply not true. They often argue that weight loss and health are simply a matter of "calories in, calories out," meaning that if you burn more calories than you consume, you will be rewarded with looser-fitting clothes and a gold star from your physician. While it's true that a calorie is a calorie, more and more studies and many scientists have come to the consensus that it is shortsighted to ignore the effects of different calorie *types* on the individual. You could, for example, decide to take in your entire day's share of calories via candy bars. But you'll pay a hefty price in terms of vitality, not to mention your teeth, compared to those who opted for a balance of lean meats, whole grains, vegetables, and healthy fats.

That's why the PrayFit Diet calorie pie chart consists of three equal slices—33-33-33—each representing a balanced and proportional dose of the three macronutrients that are absolutely crucial for good health: carbohydrates, protein, and fat. The focus is on whole foods and clean eating. I'm here to tell you that if any diet warns that an entire group of whole foods is unhealthy or off-limits (say, no fruit or no fat), be wary.

While the total amount of calories you consume on PrayFit is important, the degree to which you are able to look, feel, and actually be healthy is largely determined by the choices you make within each category and how these ratios are balanced within your total caloric intake. This type of balance is more sustainable—which means more weight lost over time—because it doesn't require drastic cuts in any one type of food. Eating in balance means that you get the benefit of a wide variety of nutritional sources without having to eliminate any.

Eating a variety of macronutrients ensures that you are taking in a well-balanced diet that provides adequate amounts of quality protein for repair and regeneration of tissues (especially muscle tissue), healthy sources of carbohydrates for steady energy, and healthy fats for proper brain function, cardiovascular health, and joint function. Taken together, this leads to marked improvements in body composition and key health markers such as cholesterol, blood pressure, and blood sugar. Combined with regular exercise, this type of approach to nutrition can also lend itself to greater strength gains and muscular endurance. Need further convincing? This diet can limit inflammation and reduce the risk of certain cancers by acting favorably on key genes. And you can do all of this without the mathematical deftness of a Harvard scholar.

The research further bears out the virtue of balance. And the man behind the charts, studies, and focus groups is one of the nation's foremost experts on nutrition as it pertains to body composition. My good friend Jim Stoppani, PhD, a PrayFit contributing expert whose dedicated examination of the existing research on the concept of equal macronutrients forms the backbone of this diet, believes that the science simply hammers home what common sense and biblical mandates have already spelled out.

Research shows that when protein and carbs are eaten in equal amounts, brain function is optimized, allowing you to be more efficient at work and on all cognitive tasks. This is due to the fact that such a diet better maintains steady blood glucose and insulin levels throughout the day. This will make you much less of a candidate for disorders such as type 2 diabetes, cardiovascular disease, and other weight-related maladies that cost Americans in excess of $190 billion in medical costs annually.

Studies also show that when these three macronutrients are eaten in equal quantities and in proper amounts, in conjunction with a proper exercise program, fat loss is enhanced, while important muscle tissue is spared or improved. That's because all three macronutrients play separate but crucial roles in the maintenance of muscle.

† If you are too low on carbohydrate—your body's preferred and primary fuel source—you will lack the energy to engage in, or recover from, activities that you enjoy. With low-carb diets you also tend to miss out on getting ample phytonutrients (see sidebar on page 36) and vitamins from fruit and whole grains.

† Going with a prolonged low-fat approach robs your joints of crucial support and can lead to greater inflammation and fat retention.

† If you opt to cut out too much protein, your muscles will lack the building blocks they require for improved shape, size, or performance, meaning that a loss of lean muscle—and consequently an increase in fat—is almost inevitable.

Because this diet also reduces inflammation in the body, it further promotes fat loss. This is due to the fact that when inflammation is high in the body—whether as a result of stress, poor nutrition, or exercise—certain chemicals known as cytokines are released that can influence fat gain. Compounding that bit of good news is that this type of eating is infinitely more sustainable than most prepackaged diets that are floating around on the market. What does that mean for you? Steady weight loss over a much longer time frame and the ability to keep it off without resorting to dietary dramatics. This is, without question, a much healthier and more productive way to meet the biblical expectations of stewardship of our bodies.

IN DEFENSE OF BALANCE

The concept of eating your macronutrients in equal proportions may seem contradictory to those who have been brought up in the school of caloric equality. Getting one-third of your day's calories from carbohydrates, it has been argued, may not be enough;

you may hear suggestions that up to 65 percent of your daily calories should come in the form of carbohydrates. Some may also be inclined to claim that so many calories from protein can be detrimental to your health. And there are others who claim that any kind of dietary fat should be avoided at all costs. But anecdotally, those eating with the 33-33-33 mantra in mind find that they enjoy the health benefits and changes to body composition without all that pesky diet-fueled despair. So what is the reality?

Carbohydrate: Less Is More

At 33 percent of your daily caloric intake, your PrayFit Diet requirement of carbohydrates provides enough quality fuel to get you through your day and prevents the type of excess that can lead to weight gain.

Claims that we need a greater percentage of daily calories from carbohydrates seem to ignore the fact that our bodies, built for survival, can function optimally under conditions that nutritional idealists might consider adverse. In a carb-deprived state, our bodies readily convert protein and fat into carbs (read: energy) when needed. This means that even if you reduce your overall carbohydrate intake, your body has a built-in safety net that it can call upon for hitting the gym or coaching your kid's soccer team.

Conversely—and perhaps tragically—the body can convert excess carbs or poor carb choices into fat quite easily. If you're not sufficiently active, too many calories from any source are a surefire bet for weight gain and other health issues, but carbohydrates, in particular, make the jump from macronutrient to fat cells in a hurry. And carb type is incredibly important because some carbs, those with a lower glycemic index (GI) rating, are digested at a much slower rate (more on this in Chapter 3), meaning that they have a much smaller impact on blood sugar and are less likely to threaten your weight-loss efforts.

Plus, higher-carb diets—those that go up to the aforementioned 65 percent threshold—have been shown by the same body of research to increase the activity of disease-causing genes in the body, while also increasing body-wrecking inflammation.

During your first thirty-three days on PrayFit, you'll start to learn how your body works and feels at a healthy 33 percent carb balance. By giving your body enough carbs to do its job—but not so many carbs that this fuel turns to fat—you'll start to turn it into the leaner, more efficient machine it was meant to be.

Protein: Higher by Design

Higher protein consumption has been demonized by some as either an unhealthy practice reserved for the guys in the weight room or a fad diet that can damage kidneys and doesn't lead to long-term weight loss. And it's true that while a lot of high-protein/low-carb diets (the so-called bacon-and-cheeseburger eating plans) may help you lose weight in the short term, they are notoriously hard to stay on for the long term, not to mention unhealthy.

Lost in the hysteria over the potentially damaging effects of higher protein consumption are the countless studies to the contrary—and the often underplayed dangers of consuming far too little protein, which is actually much more common.

While there is no reliable evidence affirming the health risks of protein, there is quite a bit of literature that elevates protein to king of the macronutrients. One recent review of protein consumption found that eating 1 gram per pound of body weight per day—or about 150 grams for a 150-pound person—is beneficial for building muscle and strength. This is vital, considering that we lose 3 to 8 percent of our total muscle mass per decade, or close to 1 percent per year, as we age. And since muscle is metabolic tissue, meaning it burns calories even while at rest, holding on to as much of it as you can helps you stave off weight gain while keeping you strong and more resistant to injuries.

And when it comes to overall impact on body composition, protein is something of a miracle food source. It is incredibly slow to be digested, which means that when it's eaten with other foods, it ensures a steadier supply of energy while preventing damaging upswings in blood sugar.

Multiple studies affirm protein's ability to help you get weight off and keep it off—when the right protein types are chosen in the proper quantities, of course. I'll teach you more about how to do this in Chapter 4. Those who exercise regularly will also find that adequate protein levels greatly support strength and, perhaps more important, recovery, allowing for more productive workouts as well as decreased muscle soreness.

But higher protein consumption alone isn't the key to sustained weight loss or improved performance. It is the balance of the macronutrients that provides the true impetus for gradual, continuous change and the downregulation of genes that trigger inflammation and disease. By equalizing your protein input at about 33 percent of your total calories on PrayFit, you'll be able to get all the positive benefits of this vital macronutrient while not letting it overwhelm your plate.

Fat: Eat It to Lose It

For a while, fat was public enemy number one in the American diet. The prevailing wisdom was that excessive fat in the body and blood can lead to increased disease as well as weight gain. The disease fears are not without merit, since high-fat indulgences such as fried fast foods are associated with higher levels of heart disease. And those who worry about dietary fat affecting the scale are justified in their concern—at 9 calories per gram, fat holds more than double the digestive danger as carbs and protein, which weigh in at 4 calories per gram.

But fats—like calories themselves—are not all created equal. The fat calories that you take in from a double cheeseburger, for example, have a different impact on the body than a similar amount of fat calories from nuts, seeds, avocados, or olive oil. The trans fats from that burger will surely cost you another notch on that belt sooner or later, whereas the polyunsaturated fats from a helping of almonds can boost heart health, activate fat-burning genes, and help to prevent certain cancers—all at the same caloric cost.

So how much is too much? When in doubt, ask the lab coats. The Malmö Diet and Cancer Study reported that individuals receiving more than 30 percent of their total daily energy from fat and more than 10 percent from saturated fat did not have increased mortality. Research out of Loma Linda University in California concluded that a higher-fat diet consisting of 39 percent fat (mostly from healthy fats such as almonds) and 32 percent carbohydrates resulted in a 56 percent greater fat loss than a diet composed of 53 percent carbs and only 18 percent fat. Put another way, you've got to eat fat to beat fat. You just need to be smart about how you choose your menu within the PrayFit Diet's 33 percent protocols. And we'll show you how.

BEYOND THE RATIOS

As simple as it is to eat carbs, protein, and fat in equal proportions, there are other nutritional strategies that can and should be implemented in order to maximize results—not just for the month but for the next year or five years. Based on slow-digested foods, fast metabolism, and long-term sustainability, the PrayFit Diet capitalizes on existing science as well as biblically sound nutritional balance that you can access in perpetuity to help you better care for the body that carries the soul.

Maybe you'll be able to lose twenty pounds on the thirty-three-day diet you'll find on the pages that follow. My exclusive list of clients as well as countless readers at PrayFit.com have lost a great deal of weight, although that's not the only benchmark I'd like you to use to track your progress. Do you feel healthier? Stronger? More able to take on the challenges ahead—challenges to your diet, your life, and your faith? And can you parlay that newfound knowledge and confidence into a loss of forty or fifty pounds in a year if medically necessary? Absolutely. Here's why.

FITNESS BY THE NUMBERS

3–8	Average percentage of muscle loss per decade in inactive adults
1	Percentage of lean muscle loss, per year, in those over age forty-five
37	Percentage of American adults who are physically inactive
8	Total percentage of the U.S. population (estimated) that lives with diabetes
285	Number, in millions, of people worldwide affected by diabetes (over 90 percent of these cases are of the more preventable type 2 variety)
300,000	Estimated number of obesity-related deaths in the United States each year
76	Percentage of Christian clergy found to be overweight or obese (compare this figure with 61 percent for the general population)

Sources: American College of Sports Medicine, *Senior Journal,* Fitness.gov, American Diabetes Association, National Institutes of Health, Duke Divinity School

---

SLOW FOODS, FAST RESULTS

Altering your menu for the better is an exercise that anyone can benefit from. But with a nutritional plan that omits very little in terms of food groups, you may wonder how you can experience the type of change in body composition I'm promising. How can you lose twenty pounds in thirty-three days if you're eating all kinds of foods? The first way is focusing on healthy, delicious foods that are slower to be digested.

We mentioned above that carbs alone are not the enemy—your body runs on the fuel they provide. Rather, certain types of carbs are hindering our collective effort to lighten the burden on pews everywhere.

When you guzzle down a sugar-laden soft drink, it touches off a rapid and catastrophic cascade of events in your body. That sugar—and there's lots of it—is a form of carbohydrate and is digested very quickly by the body, drastically increasing blood sugar levels, which in turn causes the hormone insulin to spike. Insulin is a functional protein in the body that actually signals the body to store fat for energy, playing to your body's inner self-preservationist. A trick to staying lean, then, is learning how to avoid these huge insulin dumps.

I'll show you how you can lose big by eating slow. By "slow," I'm not talking about some arbitrary number of chews per bite of food, or taking breaks between mouthfuls. Instead, we're talking about food types. The PrayFit Diet features foods that are digested slowly—namely, those that are high in complex carbohydrates, fiber, and/or lean protein.

Complex carbs such as vegetables, brown rice, and oatmeal are digested slowly and therefore have a much lower glycemic (blood sugar) impact than other carb sources such as sugary sodas, candy, white potatoes, and white rice. As a result, complex carbs are more filling and provide more nutritive value than many of the foods that are mainstays in American families' cupboards.

And protein is more important in this regard than you may think. Protein is much slower to digest than many carb sources, so consuming them together—or even protein alone, as a snack—serves two purposes. First, the constant influx of protein keeps your body working harder to digest food and provides the building blocks for muscle repair from workouts. Second, the presence of protein only further slows the digestion of carbs that you consume. The impact of foods with a higher glycemic index rating—foods that are broken down into glucose faster—will be minimized when consumed with good lean sources of protein such as beef, fish, chicken, or pork.

And though it's become more of a buzzword in diet books, fiber actually holds great value when it comes to slowing digestion. I'll touch on fiber in greater detail later, but keeping your fiber levels adequate helps to steady blood sugar levels, which maintains energy at a constant level throughout the day. This also prevents the onset of ruthless cravings that may occur with other deprivation-based diets. The PrayFit Diet is full of fiber-rich food options—think flaxseed, oatmeal, almonds, broccoli, and carrots—and helps you become a label-savvy shopper to make sure that you have an ample supply of this slimming stuff in your pantry year-round.

REVVING METABOLISM

The old "calories in, calories out" philosophers were right about one thing: burning more calories than you take in is a surefire way to lose weight. But that caloric burn doesn't have to end with the last rep in today's workout. By making some adjustments to the way you eat, you can naturally enhance your body's metabolism—its ability to convert food to fuel—helping your body to burn more calories even while parked in the pew at Sunday service.

Three meal-replacement shakes a day and a sensible dinner? Not here. While it may sound sensible to simply eat less food or to eat less often if you want to lose weight, that's just not the case. And if you've ever tried to "eat less," then you know how difficult that is. We are not meant to eat until our buttons pop off, but we're certainly not meant to live in a state of deprivation.

Provided that you're making sound food choices—which the

PrayFit Diet teaches you to do—it is more prudent to eat more frequently. That's a truth that bears repeating: if you want to see significant, long-term changes to your health and body composition, eat more frequently. Today, according to the latest research, more than 68 percent of adults are overweight or obese, with a full 33 percent falling into the latter category.

Research and a bit of common sense point to the fact that smaller, more frequent meals can produce more weight loss. For starters, eating more often is a metabolism-boosting habit. The more often your digestive system is called upon to convert food into energy (that is, digest stuff), the more often it will be using energy. These meals and snacks, however, are necessarily smaller—if you're shooting for, say, 1,800 calories per day, it wouldn't make sense to take in 1,000 calories with a massive burrito at lunch. Also, eating too much at one sitting puts a heavy strain on your digestive system. Only so much can be put to work for energy at one time, leaving the rest to take up residence in your body in the form of fat. Overeating at one sitting can also rob you of precious energy as you fall victim to the inevitable drops in blood sugar that follow.

The PrayFit Diet calls for three meals per day and snacks, each helping you to adhere to the basic principles of variety and balance I've talked about. Eating so often, even though it may seem counterintuitive, is akin to throwing fresh kindling on your metabolic fire every few hours just to keep it hot and burning bright. The PrayFit Diet shows you how to eat *more* (that is, more often) to lose more. And the inclusion of a great variety of foods— a key principle in the PrayFit Diet—allows you to do so without getting bored.

The PrayFit Diet, despite the absence of overwhelming restrictions, will still result in a lower calorie intake than some are used to. And because we are hardwired for survival, prolonged bouts of caloric deficits—however slight—can sometimes backfire. Our bodies adapt and may begin to hold on to more body fat out of sheer survival instinct. To combat this, the PrayFit Diet includes sporadic "cheat" meals, when I'll encourage you to increase caloric intake. This serves to jump-start your metabolism, allowing the PrayFit Diet to continue to work for you when you return to more structured eating.

Science dictates that the body will only change to the degree that you stress it. In keeping with that rationale, combining this type of metabolic eating with the exercise principles described at PrayFit.com will only increase your rate of weight loss.

Having a faster metabolism is absolutely within reach for those who follow the principles laid out in the PrayFit Diet.

LONG-TERM SUCCESS

Here is where the PrayFit Diet truly sets itself apart from others that you may have tried. Where other diets play to deprivation and desperation, this one calls for abundance and ongoing progress.

Because the PrayFit nutritional guidelines are built upon balance—and the research that supports it—you don't ever have to cycle off this meal plan or drastically alter it to accommodate scale stagnation. The information that you find on these pages will be as useful ten years from now as it is today.

The PrayFit Diet doesn't encourage the extraction of your sweet tooth, nor does it champion rapid weight loss at the expense of overall health. Eating your macronutrients in equal proportions facilitates weight loss, not by steering you in the direction of the drastic but by returning you to the way that you were intended to eat in the first place.

Even if you possess a basic knowledge of sound nutrition—fruits, veggies, lean meats, and so on—this more prescriptive road map eliminates the guesswork. By teaching you what a properly proportioned plate should look like, as well as the value it holds for leaner living, the PrayFit Diet allows you to feed yourself and your family without the burden of scales, calculators, or complicated formulas. The Lord didn't intend for us to fret over every single calorie in the way that other fad diets would have you believe.

Of course, some nutritional extremes may be immediately gratifying, making good on promises that you'll lose ten pounds or more in a week. What they don't tell you is that these "cleanses" and "crashes" are simply leaching your body of water while depriving you of key nutrients. After that first week or two, where do you go? Bereft of energy and desperate for sugar, many dieters lose traction at this point. Research shows that at any given time, 50 percent of American women and 25 percent of American men are on a diet of some kind. Nearly 95 percent of these people gain the weight back—and sometimes more—within one to five years. Maybe at some point you've been one of these people who resolve to lose weight without first making the lifestyle changes required for long-term success.

On these pages, what you'll find is less a "diet" than a prescription for healthy living. Some will be amazed at how simple the required changes are—reaching for different carb sources, snacking more often, and so on—and that's a good thing. Subtlety breeds sustainability and discipline creates dependence, particularly when it comes to eating habits. And those who find this type of eating to be a challenge will soon discover that the increased energy levels and better-fitting clothing are well worth the modest stretch.

There is also a spiritual tug for physical activity that is palpable, undeniable, and demonstrable within Scripture. John the Baptist jumped in his mother's womb when a pregnant Mary walked into the room. Shepherds dropped their tools and sprinted to see the newborn king. And years later, friends of a crippled man lifted him up and through the roof to be healed by Jesus. Then and now, there's just something about Him. He *moves* people. John *jumped*, shepherds *sprinted*, and friends *lifted*. And when your body is fueled better, it wants to move more, meaning that this meal plan is not just about consumption—it's about inspiration. How much more likely would you be to walk regularly with your spouse, roughhouse with your children, or return to a sport you used to love if you had the energy? If your joints felt a little better in the morning? If you found yourself stronger and more alert than you had in years past? He designed these bodies to move, and when you follow the basic tenets of this plan, you are much more likely to do that on a regular basis. And once regular, dedicated activity is part of your weekly routine, there's no limit to the changes you can make both in your body and in the world around you—in His name.

THE 33 BREAKDOWN

On the PrayFit Diet you will eat approximately 33 percent of total calories from protein, 33 percent from carbohydrates, and 33 percent from fat each day. Your goal will be to eat about 150 grams of protein, 150 grams of carbohydrates, and 75 grams of fat. This comes out to about 12 calories per pound of body weight (for a 150-pound person), or about 1,800 calories. While I've based these guidelines on a 150-pound person, in fact these dietary guidelines will work for you if you weigh anywhere from 130 to 250 pounds. (The recommendations hold throughout this weight range because of how it will affect a person at the higher end of that scale, who is perhaps carrying more body fat.)

The nutrient density of the foods prescribed in the PrayFit Diet allow you, regardless of your weight, to feel infinitely better while simultaneously working toward a particular number on the scale. Too many of our diets are heavy on empty-calorie sources—foods that are laden with too much fat, sugar, or sodium to have any positive impact on vitality. Similarly, a diet that is too restrictive deprives you of the energy needed to work, walk, or witness. By hovering around 1,800 power-packed calories, with an equal portion coming from each of the macronutrients, you'll have enough fuel stored away to tackle whatever activities you'd like, but not so much that it would lead to unwanted weight gain. Did I mention that I'm a big fan of balance?

WHAT TO DO IF YOUR BODY WEIGHT FALLS OUTSIDE THE 130–250-POUND RANGE

The reason I use 130 to 250 pounds as the range for starting body weight is that 1,800 well-balanced calories can provide energy for the day while still allowing for healthy, sustainable weight loss.

† *Those who are at the top end of the range,* 250 pounds or more, will benefit by reining in calories to this more tempered, balanced caloric goal. Most—but not all—readers in the heavier range have likely taken some liberties with their calorie intake, and getting a consistent 1,800 per day will help bring weight off quickly. However, the transition to this slightly more restricted calorie count can be tough at first. If need be, in the first few weeks you can allow yourself to go above the 1,800-calorie marker by no more than 500 calories, provided that you keep your calories in balance. But you will have to make sure that those 500 calories fall within the prescribed parameters of the overall diet. In other words, you will have to have those 500 calories equally divided among protein, fat, and carbs. This amounts to 167 calories from each, or 42 grams each of protein and carbs and 18.5 grams of fat. (Remember: every gram of protein has 4 calories; every gram of carbohydrate has 4 calories; every gram of fat has 9 calories.) The best way to take in those calories healthfully is by implementing well-timed snacks throughout the day or before bedtime. There are several snacks listed in the weekly meal plans, which begin on page 127.

† *If you are lighter than 130 pounds,* 1,800 calories may seem a bit much at first, particularly since the focus is on foods that are digested more slowly. If you find yourself feeling overly full, simply eliminate one or both snacks outlined in the meal plans. However, do not reduce your intake below 1,200 calories.

Whether you fall above or below the weight ranges listed, an increase in activity—and the move toward an ideal body weight—will help you make the most of 1,800 calories, forever.

How hard is this nutritional plan compared to others? By simply getting equal caloric amounts of carbs, protein, and fat at every meal or snack throughout the day, you can easily meet the requirements of the PrayFit Diet. So what does a day look like on the PrayFit Diet? Probably a lot tastier and diverse than you think.

Prayfit Menu Sample Day

Breakfast

1 cup nonfat Greek yogurt

2 tablespoons sliced almonds

1 tablespoon ground flaxseed

1 cup berries

Calories: 392

Total Fat: 16 g

Saturated Fat: 1 g

Carbohydrate: 38 g

Protein: 31 g

Sodium: 95 mg

Cholesterol: 0 mg

Fiber: 9 g

Lunch

3 ounces deli turkey

1 slice Swiss cheese

3 slices avocado

Sliced tomato

2 slices Ezekiel bread

Calories: 459

Total Fat: 17 g

Saturated Fat: 5 g

Carbohydrate: 42 g

Protein: 33 g

Sodium: 1,748 mg

Cholesterol: 87 mg

Fiber: 7 g

Snack

¼ cup hummus

10 baby carrots

Calories: 170

Total Fat: 9 g

Saturated Fat: 1 g

Carbohydrate: 21 g

Protein: 4 g

Sodium: 312 mg

Cholesterol: 0 mg

Fiber: 5 g

Dinner

5 ounces grilled flank steak or beef tenderloin

2 cups roasted asparagus

1 ounce crumbled blue cheese

1 baked sweet potato

Calories: 601
Total Fat: 27 g
Saturated Fat: 13 g
Carbohydrate: 37 g
Protein: 54 g
Sodium: 574 mg
Cholesterol: 122 mg
Fiber: 10 g

Totals
Calories: 1,622
Total Fat: 69 g
Saturated Fat: 21 g
Carbohydrate: 139 g
Protein: 121 g
Sodium: 2,730 mg
Cholesterol: 209 mg
Fiber: 31 g

MACRONUTRIENT: The classes of chemical compounds humans consume in the largest quantities and which provide bulk energy. These are protein, fat, and carbohydrate.

PHYTONUTRIENT: Term used to describe certain organic components of plants, including antioxidants, that can promote health and longevity.

CYTOKINES: Small, cell-signaling protein molecules that encourage inflammation.

Calories Per Unit of Macronutrient
9 calories per gram of fat
4 calories per gram of carbohydrate
4 calories per gram of protein

PRAYFIT PRACTICALITY

By now, you have probably picked up on the fact that I'm not going to send you out into the wilderness to pursue some terrifying, impractical diet. I'm simply turning the spotlight on the aspects of sound nutrition that tend to get overlooked. Despite what you may read in some magazines, eating to induce weight loss or to simply enhance general health boils down to faithfulness, discipline, and stewardship. With those elements in place, the mechanics of the PrayFit Diet become even easier to abide.

We are not slaves to food. 2 Timothy 1 tells us that we have "power and love and self-control" to guide us through challenges, both in the kitchen and outside it. And when we realize that God purposefully gave us a multitude of food choices—none of which originate from the drive-through—we can begin to take advantage of what these many sources have to offer in a way that will drive us toward our ideal body weight and steer us clear of disease.

Backed by Science

By dividing your caloric intake among protein, fat, and carbs equally, you provide an instant boost to your health and turn your body into a metabolic machine. This balance has been shown to decrease systemic inflammation and reduce the risk of disease. The carbohydrates are adequate for energy, the fat is high enough and of the right type to bolster joints and aid in heart health, and the protein is high enough to support the retention of calorie-consuming lean muscle mass. The 33-33-33 balance provides everything you need and nothing you don't—it's nourishing, satisfying, and most of all sustainable. Because you're denied nothing, you won't feel the need to overeat. In the coming chapters, you'll learn how to build a perfect plate, complete with balanced, body-friendly portions, every time.

Spirit-Led Nutrition

According to 1 Corinthians 10:23, "Everything is permissible, but not everything is beneficial. Everything is permissible, but not everything is constructive." That's not to say that occasional indulgences aren't allowed, but choosing food that fuels the body—rather than food that merely satisfies cravings—is the only true way to effect demonstrable, lasting change.

When it comes to food, there's a fine line between what we desire and what we need, one that has been blurred by supersized meals, bountiful family dinners, and expansive, post-church donut spreads. But as with everything else in our walk, what we put in our body is a choice. Proverbs 25:28 reminds us that "a man without self-control is like a city broken into and left without walls."

Still, there are others who feel trapped—confined to old habits, chained to unhealthy diets, weighed down by the kind of apathy that siphons a body of vigor and vitality. They fear change, and that's natural. But the guidelines established in these pages can be followed by those who consider that "God gave us a spirit not of fear but of power and love and self-control" (2 Timothy 1:7).

Speaking of "no fear," back in 2006 I fulfilled one of my childhood dreams by sitting down for an exclusive one-on-one conversation with Sylvester Stallone. He was promoting a new product, and so my editor in chief at the time—knowing just how special the moment would be for me—sent me to chat with him. The interview was scheduled just a few months before *Rocky Balboa* would hit theaters. I remember my wife straightening my tie before I headed up to the hotel suite where I would conduct my interview with him. It was a moment I'll never forget. I even carried a copy of my master's thesis, in which I had praised *Rocky* nearly a decade earlier, so that Mr. Stallone could sign it. Sitting there, just the two of us, was both surreal and motivating, to say the least. I remember wishing that I could convey to him just how much of an influence he had been on my life. But before I could, he said something that I repeat to myself to this day. In fact, you've likely heard it repeated in commercials or motivational videos. To one of my questions, he replied: "Jimmy, in my next film, I wrote that the world ain't all sunshine and rainbows, and it will beat you to your knees and keep you there permanently if you let it. You, me, or nobody is gonna hit as hard as life. But it ain't about how hard you hit, it's about how hard you can get hit and keep moving forward. How much can you take and keep moving forward. That's how winning is done. But you gotta take the hits."

Faith. That fireproof, battle-tested, unquenchable reservoir. It's why we take the hits. Amen! It's how we move forward. It's not just the means by which we can get back to our feet when it comes to great food choices; it's the reason we try. Mustard-seed small, mountain-moving faith. Faith in Jesus. He's the reward of trust.

Anyone can choose to eat well for a time, but only by making faith the main ingredient in your commitment to healthier living will you be able to redefine your relationship with food and discover the true breadth of what your body can do when fueled properly. Now would be a good time to join me in jotting down some goals, the "God's will and good health" kind of goals.

Perhaps your doctor has indicated that you can get off blood pressure medicine if you lose fifteen pounds. Write that down. Post it somewhere as a reminder that in order for you to live abundantly and the way God intended, you need to lose weight. As a result of that diligence, you may be able to discontinue taking medication, because your body will naturally adjust to the amount of work it takes for your heart to get blood from head to toe and back again. See, writing it down is an excellent reminder that all of that happens when you achieve your weight-loss goals.

Whatever your goals are, big and small, jot them down and refer to them daily. And as you do, whisper to yourself, "God's will and good health," because here's the thing: if it's important to you, it's important to Him. He cares when you care. He cries when you cry. Your goals of health, when listed for the right reasons, are a means of praise. Just turning your heart toward accomplishing them brings Him thanks and praise. And you know what? I think the things you accomplish through the PrayFit Diet—even if those things weren't on the list—will simultaneously glorify the Lord and amaze you.

PART II

SLOW FOODS, FAST METABOLISM

3

WHAT'S SO COMPLEX ABOUT CARBOHYDRATES?

THE SIMPLE TRUTH ABOUT THE SUGAR IN YOUR DIET

"Charge that to my account," Paul told his friend Philemon. If you're unfamiliar with this biblical story, Philemon had a slave who stole from him and ran away to Rome. But when this slave met the apostle Paul, Paul showed him how to be saved. Then Paul wrote some amazing words back to Philemon. He said that this man who was once "useless to you" was useful now. And upon the slave's return to Philemon, Paul wanted his slate clean— for him to be completely forgiven and welcomed home like a brother. From thief to saint, useless to useful.

Telling that story reminds me of how forgiving the body is. Imagine the rigors of military training or the pounding the body takes during sports; isn't it amazing how it recovers and bounces back? God sure knew what He was doing, amen! He knew all the situations we would get ourselves into, and He built us able.

You know what? The body forgives not only damage from effort but also damage from the lack of it. That's right. It doesn't take long for the body to respond to better choices of food. And when you consider that our health is only a tool—a vessel to be useful in serving others—an apologetic lifestyle may be the only response. To think that God nestled forgiveness deep within our bodies. Maybe as a picture of grace for us, maybe not. But aren't we glad that taking care of ourselves is only one way to thank the Lord for seeing only our hearts?

It's because the body is so forgiving that once you begin selecting the right foods, amazing things start to happen, especially when it comes to carbohydrates. For years, carbohydrates have been the black sheep of the dieting world. But I'm going to start off this discussion with a concept that is heresy to much of the diet book establishment: *carbs are great*. Let that soak in for a minute, because I really mean it when I say it.

Carbs are not just good, they're *great*. And in more ways than one. Foods heavy in carbs tend to taste great, sure, but they're also the best possible source of fuel for your body. So when other diet books suggest that you drastically reduce or eliminate your carbohydrate consumption (your favorite foods, which provide energy) while increasing your activity level, there is little hope of sustained success. Workouts, mood, cognitive function, and general health all suffer under such a restrictive plan, which is why so many would-be dieters fall short and start swinging the scale back the other way.

Remember, we were never meant to be at the mercy of food. The line you toe on carb consumption for healthy living, then, should be one that is marked by balance and understanding, rather than deprivation and confusion. The PrayFit Diet calls for you to consume 33 percent of your day's calories (about 600 total) from this energy-rich macronutrient.

By using this key macronutrient advantageously in your

lifestyle—particularly by choosing carbs that are digested slowly—you can tackle each day head-on, as the Lord intended.

TRUTH: CARBS ARE ENERGY

As the clock ticks on throughout the day, do you ever stop to ponder where your energy comes from? Here's a hint: it's not at the bottom of that cup of java. In fact, your body derives its energy preferentially from carbohydrates.

Contrary to what physique-minded magazines may lead you to believe, carbohydrates are the body's preferred energy source and should be consumed in enough quantity to power your daily life. Your brain's gray matter is powered by the stuff, relying on carbs exclusively for fuel. Not surprisingly, those who go on ultra-low-carb diets—which are higher in fat, a far less efficient source of energy—end up feeling sluggish and often notice marked decreases in cognitive performance and social interaction. Anecdotally, those who go without carbs for long periods of time can end up feeling depressed. Can I have a show of hands from those who have ever, in the midst of a sugar-deprived haze, "eaten their feelings" out of a box of chocolate?

A lack of carbohydrate is also highly detrimental to those who are increasing activity to match what they perceive as healthier eating. In their well-intended effort to improve body composition, those in the low-carb crowd end up finding that they cannot sustain the level of exercise required to change the body at a satisfactory rate. "I haven't had carbs for a week, so why have I not lost any weight?" they ask. Often to blame is a series of substandard workouts that are the result of inadequate energy.

Of course, those workouts may not *feel* that way, but without enough of the right energy at your disposal, and because your muscles (just like your brain) rely on stored carbohydrate for fuel, it's incredibly difficult to train harder or longer. And since progression—forcing your body to do more each time you train—is the cornerstone of change, people are quickly discouraged by the results of training on a low-carb diet.

That discouragement is compounded by the negative feelings that are commonplace when you get a case of the low-carb crankies. "If this hasn't worked by now," you may think, "it's not going to work ever! Pass the french fries." You can see why yo-yo dieting has become so commonplace.

It may not surprise you to learn that carbohydrate consumption results in the release of the feel-good hormone serotonin. So if you go without carbs for a while, as is often recommended in weight-loss diets, your body gets kind of nostalgic and begins to crave them. Consequently, when you consume carbs, not only does it taste good but it *feels* good. (Nodding are those of you who have ever been left wondering what happened to the pizza that was just in front of you.) That's the serotonin talking. A better bet is to steady out your carb consumption with sources that are digested more slowly, so that your brain never feels the need to go into survival mode. That's what the PrayFit Diet does.

You may feel like you want carbs all the time, but that's because your body *prefers* carbs as its fuel source. When your body is forced to go without, it goes on the hunt for alternative fuel sources to convert into energy, which is a much less efficient process. A better strategy is to have the right stuff on hand, right when your body needs it. Doing it this way will not only preserve your sanity but also ensure that you are adequately fueled for life.

SLOW DIGESTION, FAST RESULTS

With the PrayFit Diet, you won't eradicate carbs. You'll just become more discerning when it comes to the carbs you put on your plate or in your glass. What many people don't realize is that not all carbs are created equal. Within the vast (and tasty) legion of carbohydrate-rich foods on this planet, there exist different types, simple and complex, and each has a distinct impact on overall body composition.

Simple carbohydrates are the ones that you are probably the most enamored with. Unfortunately, most of these happen to be the worst for your overall health, energy, and waistline. Simple carbs are those that are broken down quickly by the body and used for energy. That may not sound too bad, but when sugars (simple carbs) are digested quickly, this triggers the release of insulin in the body, which causes your body to store fat. Not good. Sugary sodas, many breakfast cereals, candy, white bread, white potatoes, and white-flour tortillas are all loaded with these rapid sugars, spelling disaster for those who may not know the difference.

There are, however, healthier sources of faster-digesting simple carbs, so I don't advocate cutting them out entirely. But think carefully about which ones you select. Foods such as milk and some fruits are technically simple carbs, but these nutrient-dense foods provide other benefits, so they can be a healthy part of your 33 percent daily carb intake—within reason. Milk, for example, is rich in protein, which supports muscle recovery, and calcium, which bolsters bone strength. Fruit is generally high in fiber, which makes it ideal for keeping blood sugar in check. But it consists primarily of fructose, a form of sugar that must first travel to the liver, where it can be converted into glucose for use by the body. This takes time, of course, and results in a much less significant impact on your blood sugar. However, if your liver is stocked with glycogen—stored blood sugar—the fructose can be readily converted into fat, which is not what you want. This is why, most of the time, fruit consumption should be limited to earlier in the day.

Complex carbohydrates, on the other hand, are digested very slowly by the body and provide a steady dose of energy along the way. These foods, which include oatmeal, whole grains, and brown rice, are usually replete with fiber, vitamins, and minerals, making them something of a gold mine for those looking for an instant, noticeable upgrade in energy levels. These foods are lower on the glycemic index (GI), which serves as a measure of how fast blood sugar levels rise after consumption. Simple carbs turn to sugar quickly and cause a spike in the blood sugar—they typically rate very high on the GI. Complex carbs are processed by the body more slowly, so they provide sustained energy rather than a quick boost. The rule of thumb: the lower the GI rating, the better the food choice.

But just in case you don't have smartphone access to listings of where foods are on the glycemic index, there are some other ways you can quickly discern whether or not a food product is good or bad for you in this department: check the label. Foods that are higher in fiber are a plus—the Mayo Clinic says that if you take in 3 grams or more of fiber per serving, then you're in the right ballpark. Total carbohydrate is important as well, but you can basically lower that number by however many grams of fiber are present. If a product has 20 grams of total carbohydrates in a serving, for example, but a total of 5 grams of fiber, then your net carb intake is 15 grams. You'll also want to stay away from products that are higher in sugar—such as pastries, sodas, and ice cream—as sugar has a higher impact on blood sugar and therefore on your weight.

The PrayFit Diet will call for mostly low-GI foods. Oatmeal, vegetables, legumes, and other fiber-laden carbs will be the order of the day, allowing you to get the fuel you need without causing unnecessary spikes in blood sugar. Research from Loughborough University found that when subjects ate low-GI carbohydrates at breakfast and lunch, they had lower insulin and glucose levels and burned more fat throughout the day than when they consumed high-GI carbohydrates early in the day. In other words, it's a good idea to eat carbs—just more of the right kind. *Slow digestion equals fast results.*

COMPLEX CARB ALL-STARS

Try adding a few of these high-fiber, complex carb foods into your diet, to get the most bang for your dietary buck.

Oatmeal

There are few foods that are better to start your day with than oatmeal. Research shows it helps to lower cholesterol levels, blood pressure, and blood glucose levels, setting you up for success for the rest of the day. These claims have been affirmed by the Academy of Nutrition and Dietetics, the American Heart Association, and the U.S. Food and Drug Administration.

Ezekiel 4:9 Bread and Tortillas

Named for the passage in the Bible that advises taking grains and legumes, mixing them together, and making bread that contains no flour, Ezekiel bread and tortillas are a mix of organic sprouted whole grains such as wheat, millet, spelt, and barley, and legumes such as lentils and soybeans. As a result, Ezekiel bread and tortillas are a great source of slowly digested, low-impact carbs and complete protein. These nutritional gems can be found at health food chains such as Whole Foods, Mother's, and Trader Joe's, although many major supermarkets are starting to carry Ezekiel products as well.

Quinoa

Quinoa is a seed, not a grain. That might surprise you, but this seed, which has crept onto more and more dinner plates in recent years, is a powerful source of healthy carbs. It's gluten-free, quick-cooking, and a great source of iron. It has twice the protein of brown rice. And, like Ezekiel bread and tortillas, quinoa is a complete protein, meaning it contains all of the essential amino acids. (Complete protein is usually only found in animal products.)

Broccoli

"Jimmy, eat your broccoli." I used to shiver when Mom would say this. But not so much anymore. Turns out broccoli packs an amazing punch. An excellent source of fiber, it's also extremely low in saturated fat and cholesterol. Packed with wonderful vitamins, including A, E, and K, broccoli is also a good source of protein.

Sweet Potatoes

My favorite on the list, sweet potatoes are loaded with potassium and vitamin B_6, and they're rich in beta-carotene. So don't let the name fool you—sweet potatoes are an excellent and healthy source of complex carbohydrates.

A 2007 study from the National Taiwan College of Physical Education found that when eight male runners ran to exhaustion after eating a meal of slow-digesting carbs (consisting of Kellogg's All-Bran cereal, skim milk, peaches, apples, and apple juice), they ran for more than seven minutes longer than when they ate a meal of fast-digesting carbs (consisting of Kellogg's Corn Flakes, skim milk, white bread, jam, a glucose drink, and water) beforehand. The slower-digesting carbs lead to steadier streams of available energy.

HOW TO EAT CARBS ON THE PRAYFIT DIET

Though I've said a lot about the value of carbs, on the PrayFit Diet your carbohydrate consumption will still be kept modest. Remember, balance with the other macronutrients—protein and fat—is the key to reaping all the benefits in terms of weight loss, energy levels, and performance.

Each day, you will consume approximately one-third of your day's calories from carbs—600 calories, or about 150 total grams of carbohydrate. What would that look like? Here's a snapshot. Over the course of a day, that might shape up to include a cup of cooked oatmeal, two slices of bread, a piece of fruit, half a cup of brown rice, and a large veggie salad. There are more examples of how to build healthy carbs into your day in our meal plans, beginning on page 125.

This tempered approach ensures that you are getting enough of this ideal fuel source without going overboard. At 33 percent of your day's calories, your carb consumption will be plenty adequate for whatever your workout schedule includes, while still keeping your brain and body performing at optimal levels. This helps to ensure that your body is able to shed fat steadily *without* driving you mad from deprivation.

But better body composition isn't the only reason to keep your carb counts within reason. Researchers at the Norwegian University of Science and Technology found that those who ate high-carb diets for six days had a significant increase in systemic (total body) inflammation, which raises the risk for other maladies such as cardiovascular disease, type 2 diabetes, cancer, and dementia. So you'll be losing weight today, and you'll be safeguarding your health for tomorrow, too.

THE CARB KEY: FIBER

I've already talked about the importance of choosing complex carbohydrates. And one phenomenal way to find good carb sources is to look for those that are high in fiber. Ah, yes . . . fiber. In full disclosure, it's the first item my eyes scan for when shopping. My wife will tell you, when I grab something off the shelf, I'm trolling for grams of fiber. Over the last few years, I've come to appreciate beyond measure the importance of fiber in our diet. The positive consequences of fiber-rich foods are innumerable.

More than just a dietary catchword, fiber is a wonder food that most people can stand to have more of. Basically, it is a form of complex carbohydrate that can slow the breakdown and digestion of many foods we eat. That is a desirable effect because, again, it reduces those pesky swings in blood sugar and insulin. This means that food stays in your system longer, extending the energy release that food provides. And because of this digestion slowdown, fiber has a satiety effect, making you feel fuller longer. This means that you are less likely to go reaching for unhealthy snacks in the hours that follow a high-fiber meal.

Because of its effects on the digestive system, fiber counts actually work to offset carb counts in food. In other words, if you eat something that has 15 carbohydrate grams and 5 grams of fiber, you're only getting 10 grams of net carbohydrates. So a steady intake of fiber-rich foods throughout the day is an easy way to stay full, keep energy levels up, and limit the potential glycemic impact of the foods you do take in.

There are two types of fiber worth considering: soluble and insoluble. *Soluble fiber*, which is easily dissolved in water, is found in foods such as citrus fruits, oats, legumes, and barley, and it keeps cholesterol levels in check while stabilizing blood sugar. *Insoluble fiber*, which is not easily dissolved, is found primarily in nuts, seeds, whole grains, and veggies and possesses huge benefits for digestive health—that means more nutrients make it where they're supposed to and you are less likely to suffer intestinal distress, dysfunction, or disease.

Yes, fiber . . . fiber . . . fiber. If there's one thing I know, and one thing I need you to know, it's that fiber is critical to our health. From digestion to eating and feeling satisfied and fuller longer, it's my wonder food. I urge you to make the conscious effort and ensure you include the healthy fiber choices I recommend within these pages. My sense of urgency for fiber sources was born out of my personal infirmities, some of which doctors say I inherited from Mom and Dad, but *all* of which I'm conquering by implementing the PrayFit Diet, just as I'm recommending you do.

And I am serious about my fiber. I literally take it with me everywhere I go. Recently, my wife and I had the privilege to travel to an exotic, private island of one of my clients. True paradise. But one thing that made its way into my luggage and all the way across the Atlantic was my fiber stash. I wasn't taking any chances. Other than our relationship with God, nothing, and I mean nothing, is more important than our health.

A large review of studies published in 2011 in the British Medical Journal found that high-fiber diets were associated with a lower risk of colorectal cancer. Another study found that those who ate a diet rich in fiber were at lower risk of cardiovascular disease, type 2 diabetes, and weight gain.

Did you catch that last part? Eating more fiber—a carb—can actually have an impact on what the scale is telling you, while providing a slew of other health benefits.

The bottom line: if there's fiber in it, you probably want it. Great sources of high-fiber goodness include berries, apples, pears, nuts, whole grains, flaxseed, oatmeal, beans, carrots, and dark green vegetables.

HIGH-FIBER FAVES

Here are a few common carb sources of healthy fiber.

Food	Serving	Fiber (carbs/serving)
Fruits		
Raspberries	1 cup	8.0 (15 grams carbs)
Pear, with skin	1 medium	6.0 (28 grams carbs)
Apple, with skin	1 medium	4.4 (25 grams carbs)
Banana	1 medium	3.1 (27 grams carbs)
Orange	1 medium	3 (15 grams carbs)

(continued on next page)

Food	Serving	Fiber (carbs/serving)
Cereals, Grains, Pasta		
Whole-wheat spaghetti, cooked	1 cup	6.3 (37 grams carbs)
Barley, pearled, cooked	1 cup	6.0 (44 grams carbs)
Bran flakes	¾ cup	5.3 (24 grams carbs)
Oat bran muffin	1 medium	5.2 (55 grams carbs)
Oatmeal, instant, cooked	1 cup	4.0 (32 grams carbs)
Legumes, Nuts, Seeds		
Split peas, cooked	1 cup	16.3 (41 grams carbs)
Lentils, cooked	1 cup	15.6 (40 grams carbs)
Black beans, cooked	1 cup	15.0 (41 grams carbs)
Lima beans	1 cup	13.2 (40 grams carbs)
Baked beans, vegetarian, cooked	1 cup	10.4 (54 grams carbs)
Vegetables		
Artichoke, cooked	1 medium	10.3 (14 grams carbs)
Green peas, cooked	1 cup	8.8 (25 grams carbs)
Broccoli, boiled	1 cup	5.1 (12 grams carbs)
Turnip greens, boiled	1 cup	5.0 (6 grams carbs)
Brussels sprouts, cooked	1 cup	4.1 (12 grams carbs)

Source: Mayo Clinic/NutritionData.com

OH, PEAR: A medium-sized pear—about the size of a tennis ball—is one of the highest-rated fruits on the fiber scale, weighing in at 6 grams per pear. And don't skip the skin—it contains fiber!

APPLE ALL-STAR: Apples are rich in pectin, a soluble fiber. Apple pectin has been shown to reduce cholesterol, control blood pressure, and lower the risk of colorectal cancers. It has also been shown to reduce the severity of diabetes.

You know, there are those who say, "Since life is so quick, why not eat up?" Well, by now you know that my reply is, "Since life is so brief, why not stay the course?" Think about it. Where does God live? He lives inside of us. Our bodies are His dwelling place. How much respect are we showing if we have a willful disregard for what certain foods—not to mention what certain *amounts* of foods—can do to our bodies? Again, this won't translate into long-lasting change unless you see healthy eating as an act of obedience.

Now, I'm not saying you can't enjoy food—because everything you're about to eat on the PrayFit Diet is delicious—but too many of our friends, siblings, parents, and kids are struggling with food-related illness. It's a battle we were never meant to fight, and one we're sure to lose unless we:

- † Bring foods into balance
- † Shop smarter
- † See the plate differently
- † Teach ourselves and our kids perfect portion control

All of which you will learn, implement, enjoy, and thrive upon with the PrayFit Diet. And besides, God didn't design us to be at the mercy of food. Let's bless His heart by taking care of ours. And nowhere does that blessing manifest itself more than when you carefully choose and time carbohydrates. Fortunately, when it comes to carbohydrates, there's no need to take an all-or-none approach.

PRAYFIT CARB SWAPS

What's in your pantry? Make these simple swaps to start maximizing the benefits you get from carbs.

White Potato vs. Sweet Potato

WINNER: SWEET POTATO

White potatoes, no matter how you eat them—fried, mashed, baked, or otherwise—are one of the tastiest, most feel-good foods that the Lord blessed us with. But a better choice would be the sweet potato. Sweet potatoes are slightly higher in fiber (3 grams vs. 2.3 for the white potato per 100-gram serving), are lower on the glycemic index, and contain more vitamins.

White Rice vs. Brown Rice

WINNER: BROWN RICE

While white rice is not necessarily bad for you, it can be higher on the glycemic index, which is not ideal for weight loss. But provided you are not dousing it in butter and other calorie-rich sauces, you're not doing too bad for yourself. However, since eating two servings or more per week of brown rice has been shown to decrease your risk of developing type 2 diabetes by 16 percent or more, brown rice holds the edge.

White Pasta vs. Whole-Wheat Pasta

WINNER: WHOLE-WHEAT PASTA

Yes, you can eat pasta—but whole-grain versions are best. This darker version of pasta offers a similar taste and texture with far more vitamins, minerals, and fiber than its traditional white counterpart. The additional fiber slows down digestion, lessening the impact on your blood sugar—if you keep the portion within reason, of course.

CARBOHYDRATE TIMING TIPS

Does *when* you eat your carbs count? The answer is sort of . . . and not really.

Again, this is a topic that's much discussed in other weight-loss books, with some diet gurus advocating no carbs first thing in the morning, and others telling you to swear off carbs after a certain time in the afternoon. PrayFit is a balanced approach, and I'm not going to push for any kind of extreme restrictions on carbs. The PrayFit Plate, after all, includes a 33 percent carb intake over the course of the day—ideally at each meal.

But consistent with what we've said earlier, the type of carbs you consume at different times of the day can have an effect on how effectively your body will allow you to lose weight. Complex carbs such as brown rice and oatmeal are almost always preferable to simple carbs such as soda and white bread, but that's especially true later in the day.

As you'll learn below, there are certain timing issues that you can and should take advantage of to ensure that these carbs are being put to work for your body instead of being left to linger at your waistline.

FAST FACT: There are two times of the day when simple carbs are less likely to impact your waistline: first thing in the morning and after a hard workout. During sleep and exercise, your body burns through stored sugars, leaving you in something of a carb deficit. At most other times of the day, excess carbs or fast-burning carbs are more likely to result in stored body fat.

Morning Carbs

Since your brain and body run on stored carbohydrate for the seven to nine hours that you are sleeping, when you wake you are in what is considered to be a carbohydrate deficit. Essentially, you have been fasting for as long as you've been asleep, and by the time the alarm shudders you out of your slumber, your body is begging for a quick refuel. That's why your breakfast is a great window for carbs.

You'll want to quickly replenish what was burned overnight, as well as tossing the right kindling on your metabolic fire for the day ahead. Most breakfasts on the PrayFit Diet will provide 40 grams or more of motor-revving, long-lasting carbohydrate fuel from sources such as oatmeal, whole grains, and fiber-rich cereals. These higher-fiber choices promote a sense of fullness, keeping you from reaching into your snack drawer at work as the morning wears on while also keeping you energized for whatever tasks lie ahead.

Immediately After a Workout

Whether you run, lift, swim, box, walk, or spin, exercise burns through carbohydrates. Your muscles rely on glycogen (stored carbs) to push through whatever you've chosen to throw at them, and after your last mile, rep, or lap, it's time to replace it. Remember, keeping your energy levels consistent—a function of regular, healthy nutrition—is an important factor in limiting over- or undereating throughout the day. And after a tough workout, replacing that lost energy is critical for that purpose.

But it's also key in recovery. Having a carbohydrate helping of 40 to 60 grams (depending on your activity level) along with 20 to 40 grams of protein after a workout will help to replace lost glycogen and trigger the hormonal responses necessary to get your body on the mend. The real changes to body composition happen during recovery, not exertion, so proper post-exercise nutrition cannot be overlooked. After a hard workout, you'll want to immediately repair muscles and replenish energy stores. The best way to do this is with an immediate infusion of lean protein and healthy carbs. A meal consisting of a chicken breast, rice, and veggies—ideally within an hour after your workout—is a safe bet to meet all requirements.

For exercise plans, tips, and videos to help you speed your results, visit www.prayfit.com.

Late Night

The PrayFit Diet is designed to help you achieve greater weight loss and vitality through consistent meals and nutritional balance. Each meal will work you toward a particular daily caloric intake at a certain macronutrient ratio (33-33-33). And while not everyone's appetite will be the same, those who have a tendency to hit the pantry after dinner and whose primary goal is weight loss should exercise additional discretion. Carbs consumed later at night, when activity level is waning, are more likely—although not certain—to be stored as body fat, which is counterproductive. If you've met your caloric goals for the day, don't let habit or even hunger pull you to the kitchen after your last meal of the day.

If you've kept your calories in check and feel the need to nosh, there are some late-night options that are better than others in the carb department. Some carrots with hummus, Greek yogurt, a handful of nuts, or a small serving of whole-grain cereal with milk are all acceptable. Consisting of mostly higher-fiber (read: more slowly digested) sources of carbohydrate and combined with protein and fats to reduce the risk of blood sugar spikes, these snacks can help if cravings come calling.

LABEL WISE: SUGAR = CARBS

While reading labels can sometimes be confusing or intimidating—food makers can "hide" particular ingredients in a number of ways—your health is still worth a peek. And when it comes to keeping yourself lean and healthy, one easy culprit to reduce by way of reading labels is sugar. Sugar is typically listed under carbohydrates, since a portion of your carb serving will likely come from sugar. The lower the sugar count, the better. A popular breakfast cereal for kids reads:

Total Carbohydrates	25 g
Dietary Fiber	3 g
Sugars	12 g

While each serving comes in at a modest 25 grams of carbohydrate, nearly half of those carbohydrate grams come from sugars. Anywhere you see sugar on a label, it is represented as a portion of the total carbohydrate count. Where it's obvious, as in this example, it's easy to pass over the product and move on to a lower-sugar option. But there are some other, more clandestine ways that food manufacturers slip sugars into our fridges and pantries.

Hidden in Plain Sight

Sugar isn't just the white stuff you put in your coffee (which you should be limiting anyway). It can also be cleverly disguised on a label. If you spy the words "syrup," "sweetener," or anything ending in "-ose," you can safely assume it to be sugar.

Sugar Alcohols

Neither sugar nor alcohol, this is a prevalent ingredient in "sugar-free" products. Sugar alcohols affect blood sugar levels less dramatically than table sugar and they won't harm your teeth, but they can cause stomach upset and bloating, and if they're consumed too often, they can derail your get-lean efforts. You know there are sugar alcohols in a product if you see any of these on the label: mannitol, sorbitol, xylitol, maltitol, maltitol syrup, galactitol, erythritol, inositol, ribitol, dithioerythritol, dithiothreitol, glycerol, or hydrogenated starch hydrolysates. If a product is labeled "sugar free" or "no added sugar," the manufacturer must show the sugar alcohol content, expressed in grams just like with normal sugar.

Like other components of the PrayFit Diet, sugar won't be completely eliminated. But as a nation, we consume far too much of it and not always by choice. By understanding how sugar is concealed on food labels, you'll be able to make smarter choices each trip to the market. Part Three provides comprehensive weekly PrayFit Diet shopping lists.

DIABETES: CAUSE FOR CONCERN

On my way to my spine surgeon a few years ago, I stood next to a man who was less fortunate than I was, because he was homeless. My heart broke. And in that moment I whispered, "Lord, help him." And then it was as if God said, "I am. You're closest." Oh, friends, it hit me like a ton of bricks: this is what our health is for. We can't be fit for fit's sake, but we can be healthy for Heaven's sake.

Two hours later, the look on my surgeon's face said it all. He proceeded to tell me that another vertebra was broken, and that I'd lose another disk in my back. The degenerative disease was eating me up. But in that moment, I knew that despite it all, my health was still a means to share Christ. I'll say it again: *Life is not about the body, but our health is a means of praise.* The more adversity weakens my muscles, the more God strengthens my message. And until life's final war with pain, I want to stand up as straight as possible and be reckless.

You know, when it comes to our health challenges, one of the most daunting dilemmas we're facing as a nation of believers is type 2 diabetes. Somebody you know and love may be battling it right now. Maybe the stranger next to you is. Maybe you are.

If so, let this be a wake-up call. One of the greatest risks of our addiction to the wrong kinds of carbohydrates is type 2 diabetes. While there are many factors associated with type 2 diabetes, including genetics, lack of sleep, and gender, lifestyle and obesity are among the main causes.

An estimated 285 million people around the globe have diabetes, and the numbers are on the rise. Sadly, because it's a condition that you can live with relatively symptom-free for years, people are failing to see cause for alarm. A new study by the Centers for Disease Control and Prevention (CDC) may change that. According to the CDC, as many as one in three Americans could be diabetic by 2050 unless action is taken.

Diabetes was the seventh-leading cause of death in 2007, and it is the leading cause of new cases of blindness among adults under age seventy-five, kidney failure, and non-accident-or-injury-related leg and foot amputations among adults. People with diagnosed diabetes have medical costs that are more than twice those of people without the disease. The total costs of diabetes are an estimated $174 billion annually, including $116 billion in direct medical costs. About twenty-four million Americans have diabetes, and one-quarter of them do not know they have it.

In the lifestyle category, those who are overweight, those who consume lots of high-sugar products, trans fats, and saturated fats, and those who don't exercise are at the greatest risk. A moderate carb intake with proper choices, the selection of healthy fats (see Chapter 5), and an increase in activity can all greatly reduce your chances of developing diabetes. In many cases, it is entirely preventable through diet and exercise. As I alluded to earlier, we are the generation most capable of living in a healthy way. When we are armed with these statistics and know the impact that poor nutrition can have on our bodies, it becomes an issue of willful neglect. Our health is a gift, and the best way we can express our gratitude is to be faithful stewards—to take every opportunity at our disposal to avoid unnecessary ailments such as diabetes.

SAD BUT TRUE: Diabetes is recognized as a global epidemic by the World Health Organization.

CARBS: 33 PERCENT OF THE PRAYFIT PLATE

Do you want abundant health? Start praying and eating with purpose. Because faith can move mountains, I believe it can do wonders with our bodies. I believe you and I were made to overcome, because God is at work in our lives. That's why we've boiled everything down to the smallest elements, the calorie, so that you can harness everything your body was built to do. And "doing" is exactly what the healthiest carb choices are phenomenal at. The body's preferred fuel source cannot be overemphasized. So absolutely pray and eat with purpose. You have mountains in life to move.

The PrayFit Diet's prescription of 33 percent of your day's calories from carbohydrate—with an emphasis on slow-to-be-digested complex carbs—helps you to optimize the benefits of this macronutrient, filling you with vigor and fortifying you against disease. It is a balanced approach to carbs—not an outright elimination of them—that will allow for more abundant living, right now.

In Chapter 4, we'll discuss how to add the next 33 percent of your diet, protein, and in Chapter 5 we'll discuss the impor-

KEY CARB TAKEAWAYS

† Carbohydrates (carbs) are the body's preferred source of energy, but they're not all created equal.

† Choose slower-to-be-digested carbs for better energy and body composition.

† Keep carb intake at 33 percent of daily calories for optimal weight loss and overall health.

† Fiber reduces the impact of carbs, helps digestion, and keeps weight off.

† Read labels: sugar equals carbohydrate.

† When it comes to carbs, timing counts, too.

tant role of fats in the PrayFit Diet. Then we'll start to put it all together and show you how to use these delicious new foods to build your PrayFit Plate, the basis of each meal during the thirty-three-day program . . . and hopefully for the rest of your life. And as we proceed, keep in mind the story of Paul and Philemon. Their agreement of a clean slate is an excellent reminder that the body is extremely forgiving. It doesn't take long for it to respond to better food choices. Start today. Start now. Clean slate, clean plate . . . freedom.

4

PROTEIN POWER

WHY MANY OF US DON'T GET ENOUGH,
AND HOW TO USE IT TO FUEL WEIGHT LOSS

Many of you may be familiar with the scene in the book of Matthew when Jesus entered the temple. What He found there didn't resemble its purpose. It didn't take Him long to overturn some tables and drive out those who mistreated His holy place. Interestingly, the very next verse says, "The blind and the lame came to Him in the temple, and He healed them."

What a picture. The Lord sees the temple being misused and mistreated, He overturns the tables, and then He heals those in need. With that image in mind, it's important for you to fully grasp that the enemy wants us to abuse the temple, this body. He wants us either to neglect it so that we can't live an abundant life or to lose perspective with vain eyes. That's why we need to ask Jesus to help us overturn some tables. He can rebuild what we've destroyed. After all, it's His temple. And that's where He heals us, the blind and the lame.

I'm hoping you're ready to overturn some tables—the breakfast, lunch, and dinner ones. You know, there are a lot of ways that we fall short of reaching our bodies' nutritional needs when trying to lose weight. As we saw in the last chapter, low-carb dieters tend to fall short of their bodies' fuel needs by restricting even healthy, complex carbs, causing blood sugar to drop and energy to flag, and making us vulnerable to unhealthy food choices. And as we'll see in the next chapter, those who opt for a low-fat approach tend to miss out on valuable omega-3 fatty acids, monounsaturated fats, and healthy doses of saturated fat that offer protection for their hearts and joints, regulate metabolism, and trigger favorable hormonal responses.

But almost universally, and regardless of the kind of diet they are on, most people tend to consume inadequate levels of protein. A 2011 study by the Centers for Disease Control and Prevention found that adults age twenty and over get only about 15 percent of their daily calories from protein. This falls well below most recommended minimums, including the recommendations in the PrayFit Diet. On PrayFit, you consume a full 33 percent of your day's calories from protein. That ratio may seem high or intimidating to many, but again, the focus is on balance. I'll teach you how to eat for power, and how ingesting more (and better) protein will stoke your metabolism for weight loss.

A 2005 study published in the *American Journal of Clinical Nutrition* found that increasing protein from 15 percent to 30 percent of total calories while bringing fat consumption into balance led to greater sustained weight loss than for those who kept protein consumption lower. Researchers had nineteen subjects go on diets consisting of 50 percent carbohydrate. Every two weeks, they varied the amount of protein and fat that subjects consumed. In the first two weeks, subjects had 15 percent of calories from protein and 35 percent from fat. In the four weeks that followed, subjects had double that amount of protein (30 percent) and 20 percent fat. And wouldn't you know it—the increased protein intake resulted in increased satiety among study participants, which led to fewer calories consumed. Put another way, eating more protein—which also suppresses your appetite for longer—is a great way to support your get-lean efforts.

Because your muscles are made of protein, getting enough of it in your diet helps to ensure that your muscles remain strong and that they function effectively. This is particularly important as we age, since we tend to lose 3 to 8 percent of our muscle mass each decade. You may not think that growing or retaining muscle is important, but one important factor to consider is the nature of muscle: it eats, constantly.

Muscle is metabolic tissue, meaning that it is burning up calories even while you rest. That's why those in the aforementioned study were more successful at losing weight. The more muscle you have, the better your body is at burning calories. This, of course, doesn't mean that you should devote yourself to an ultra-high-protein, weight-room-only lifestyle—an excess of protein won't do you much good, either. Rather, a greater focus on this important macronutrient can only serve to benefit you in both the short term and the long term.

When balanced out with the right carbs and fat sources, a diet rich in protein supports muscles, promotes fat burning, speeds recovery, and keeps us away from the vending machines at work and school.

PURPOSEFUL PROTEIN

Even those who aim for a higher-than-normal level of protein consumption can find it hard to get enough of it. Clean, lean sources of protein such as fish, beef, chicken, eggs, and turkey usually require some level of preparation, and in our increasingly busy worlds that is not always an option. But with the proper planning and the right foods at your disposal, you put yourself at much higher odds of reaching your 33 percent protein goal each day.

Below I'll make the case for exactly why protein is so important. And then I'll give you a few easy, time-saving ways to incorporate more protein into your meals. The result? If you make the effort to eat more delicious, lean protein in your diet (33 percent of calories—600 calories or 150 g), your effort will be rewarded with a leaner, healthier, and altogether more productive body. Forget about better-fitting clothes; a stronger, fitter body will allow you to physically do more in your church, community, and home.

Protein Promotes Satiety

Eating well at home is easy. You're in a familiar place, with familiar foods, all prepared to your liking and needs. Where most people get themselves into trouble is out of the house—drive-throughs, lunch trucks, and vending machines all present easy ways to satisfy hunger throughout the day. Work, school, and play dates are all riddled with nutritional land mines. One way to prevent dietary disaster later in the day is to start your day with a solid, healthy breakfast. And protein has to be a part of it.

In the previous chapter, we discussed the importance of slow-to-be-digested carb sources such as oatmeal. But there may be no better breakfast food in the area of weight management than good old-fashioned eggs. With each crack of that shell into a bowl or sizzling-hot pan, you are providing your body a much-needed punch of muscle-friendly protein while also setting yourself up for a full day of dietary restraint. First thing in the morning, your muscles are starving for amino acids—the building blocks of protein—and eggs provide a quick dose. Just one egg contains 6 grams of protein and all ten essential amino acids. Research presented at the 2012 European Congress on Obesity showed that those who ate eggs for breakfast ended up consuming fewer calories later in the day, particularly at lunch. Another study that pitted eggs against bagels as breakfast food showed similar results—eggs resulted in greater satiety and therefore fewer calories consumed later.

But this gut-filling phenomenon isn't just reserved for the breakfast table. Even though protein contains only 4 calories per gram, your body has to work very hard to digest it—and that takes time. Additional research in the journal Cell explains that protein may trigger the stimulation of mu-opioid receptors, or MORs, which then signal the stomach to release glucose, curbing appetite. Elsewhere, studies show that those on a low-protein diet—10 percent of total calories—consumed 12 percent more calories over four days than they did on a slightly higher protein intake. Translation: the more healthy protein you take in, the less likely you are to overdo it elsewhere.

To get the most out of this filling effect, the PrayFit Diet advocates having healthy protein throughout the day. To do this, you have to think beyond the chicken breast. Handfuls of nuts, string cheese, cottage cheese, and Greek yogurt are all great, protein-heavy snack options to get you from one meal to the next.

Protein Supports Weight Loss

When you consider the various snack-sized options of protein available to you, getting to that goal of 33 percent of your daily calories through protein doesn't seem so daunting. One study in the journal Nutrition and Metabolism showed that the amount of protein retained within muscle fibers was best when protein was consumed every three hours. Once you realize how easy it is to feed your body adequately in this department, you're well on your way to improving your overall physique—and you'll hold on to more muscle while continuing to lose body fat.

When you cut back on protein consumption, yes, you are reducing your overall number of calories, but you are also limiting your body's ability to build and repair muscle tissue. This is true across the board, but if you are working out as part of a weight-loss plan, protein shortages will leave you spinning your wheels. Unless you boost consumption of the other macronutrients—which, as we've shown, can lead to disastrous consequences—you're likely to be left with inadequate energy to perform effective workouts. Moreover, you will be limiting your body's ability to effectively repair muscle tissues damaged by exercise.

When you train, your body breaks down muscle fiber via tiny tears. In the sixty to ninety minutes after you exercise, protein synthesis—the process that fixes those tears and then makes them stronger for the next workout—is elevated. If you haven't consumed enough protein for the day, chances are that muscle recovery will suffer and that you will derive significantly less benefit from the sweat that you just worked up.

The good thing about workouts that include resistance is that they harness your body's metabolic furnace by focusing on this cycle of breakdown and repair. Over time, those who strengthen muscles while continuing to lose body fat have the greatest odds of continued success, because muscle burns calories. Protein aids in this process by repairing muscle quickly and more completely. As muscles are rebuilt, they improve in tone, quality, and appearance, acting favorably on your lean-tissue-to-fat ratio. This, in turn, gives you a metabolic upgrade. For every muscle fiber you tone, you force your body to burn more calories, even at rest. Those who train with resistance—even their own body weight—show higher resting metabolisms in the twenty-four to thirty-six hours following a workout than those who only engage in cardiovascular activity.

Over my career, I've had the enormous blessing of serving some of Hollywood's most popular names, including Tyler Perry, Mario Lopez, and LL Cool J, and if there's one thing that I've stressed to each of them as I helped them prepare for magazine covers, TV appearances, and movie roles, it's that they can't miss their protein. Let me rephrase that: I wouldn't *let* them miss their protein. It was my job to ensure they were at their best, and that began and ended with a healthy, balanced influx of protein. The same philosophy I use with my friends in Hollywood, I'm teaching you now.

Bottom line: Want a more active metabolism? Then you need a higher-protein approach to your daily diet.

MYTH:
PROTEIN WILL MAKE WOMEN "BULKY"

Some women are apprehensive about greater protein intake in conjunction with a regular workout program, not just for fear of unwanted calories but out of fear of adding too much muscularity. Not to worry, ladies. The type of hypermuscularity you are worried about is incredibly difficult to achieve. It is far easier for men to add muscle mass through training and diet simply due to the higher levels of testosterone they possess, but even then it takes years of progressive training and increased protein intake to achieve significant gains.

For women, adding to your protein intake during bouts of resistance training—or activity of any type, for that matter—only serves to improve the shape and quality of your muscles while also increasing your rate of fat burning. In short: more protein, better muscles, less fat.

To illustrate more benefits of protein, look outside the realm of performance. Research published in the *American Journal of Clinical Nutrition* suggests that a protein intake of 2.5 grams per kilogram of body weight—or about 1.25 grams per pound—per day for patients who were critically ill may be optimal for speedy recovery. This dose of protein, they found, was effective for patients who were on the mend and in need of more rapid muscle repair. The application for those of us just looking to shed a few pounds is more understated but equally important, because as a nation we are suffering from our own form of "critical illness": obesity.

Proper Proteins Count

Not all forms of protein are equal in their efficacy or practicality. As Paul said, while everything is permissible, not all of it is beneficial (1 Corinthians 10:23). So as much as I'd love to say that bacon and T-bones are all you need on your way to your 33 percent protein goal, that's just not the truth. Just as I recommend a balance in the total amount of protein you should consume, I also call for you to exercise balance and discretion in the types of protein you eat.

That double-patty cheeseburger that society raves about has plenty of protein (37 grams), but it is also dripping with more than a day's worth of saturated fat and sodium. Want to think smaller? Bacon contains 10 grams of protein but is weighed down by 12 grams of fat and a whopping 151 total calories . . . in a single ounce! Clearly, these are not the choices that should come to mind when you think about abundant health. When it comes to choosing the right protein source, always choose lean meats over their more thoroughly marbled, saturated-fat-rich counterparts, and avoid meats that are overly processed (this includes most deli meats) and laden with unhealthy fats or unnecessary sugars and sodium.

I've already talked about the incredible edible egg as a great protein source, but eggs have had their detractors. For years, doctors cautioned against the consumption of too many eggs, which were thought to raise cholesterol and elevate the risk of heart disease. But that thought has since abated, thanks in large part to deeper research. Studies cited by researchers at UC Berkeley point out that there has been no conclusive link between egg consumption and heart disease, except in people with diabetes. The researchers also point out that dietary cholesterol raises blood cholesterol in only about one-third of people and that a resulting rise in "good" cholesterol, or HDL, offsets any potential damage from a rise in LDL. So go ahead and put eggs back in the "safe" column.

Other proteins on the PrayFit Diet are as likely to stand up to similar scrutiny. That's because this plan is replete with protein options that are both healthy and tasty. Foods such as ground turkey, grilled chicken, flank steak, salmon, and pork chops all make the healthy-living menu, and with some spiced-up recipes thrown in, you'll never be in want of ideas for physique-friendly protein sources.

HOW TO CHOOSE THE BEST PROTEINS FOR THE PRAYFIT DIET

Protein is the most thermogenic of all three macronutrients, meaning that it requires or produces more heat (read: energy) during digestion.

Consider for a moment that for every 100 calories of protein, the body will utilize around 30 of those calories just to digest them. For every 100 calories of carbs, the body will use about 15 calories to process them. And finally, for every 100 calories of fat consumed, the body will utilize approximately only 5 for processing. It's easy to see, then, that protein is a highly metabolic food source.

Researchers at the University of Illinois at Urbana-Champaign found that women eating a higher-protein diet lost more weight over a ten-week period than a group of women on a higher-carb diet. What's notable is the percentage of weight lost that was from body fat: the protein group lost about *twice* the amount of body fat. The researchers noted that women in the high-protein group expressed a higher level of reported satiety as well.

What that means for you on the PrayFit Diet is simple: protein is your friend. With a third of your diet coming from clean, lean protein sources, you won't ever feel like you're missing out. One peek at the meal plans beginning on page 125 will be proof enough of that. But beyond the tasty, satisfying recipes that you'll dive into over the next thirty-three days, there are other ways that protein will help you reach your goals.

Protein fills. Studies show that increasing protein intake—even without reducing carb intake—increases satiety and reduces appetite. This results in fewer cravings, less overeating, and a better ability to maintain healthy habits along the way. By taking your consumption to 33 percent of your daily calories (approximately 600 calories, or about 150 grams of protein) you give yourself the best chance of keeping your fitness and health journey on track.

Protein builds. No matter how much activity you engage in every day—whether it's walking around the block or tackling your favorite at-home workout video—your muscles are stressed and broken down to varying degrees. Adequate protein consumption supplies those muscles with the building blocks they need to rebuild and repair, making you stronger for whatever comes next. This also helps you to grow or maintain lean muscle, which is important for supporting resting metabolism (calories burned while at rest).

Protein goes slow. As with complex carbohydrates, protein has a hidden superpower: it slows down digestion. It takes your body a long time to break protein down into its more usable amino acids, so when you eat it with other food—even if the other food is more likely to cause a spike in blood sugar—the delay in digestion acts in your favor. The slower the digestion, the better your body is at processing food for energy and essential functions.

Your Go-To Proteins

CHICKEN BREAST. There's a reason that you see a picture of a chicken breast with an attractive garnish on the cover of every other recipe or diet book: they are awesome. This staple protein is superlean, user-friendly, and quick-cooking, and it is also low in cholesterol and saturated fat.

FISH. If you're a fish lover, you're probably already familiar with the fact that fish provides a lighter yet wholly satisfying alternative to chicken and steak. Fish, as you might know, factor prominently in one of the most famous Bible stories: the feeding of the five thousand, which was accomplished with just two catches from the sea. What surprises most people is that fish is actually very high in fat, although most of it is healthy. You can read more about fish and how it fits into the PrayFit Diet on page 78.

EGGS. Eggs are the perfect breakfast food. While there exist volumes of research on protein and its effects on the body, there is actually quite a bit on eggs as well. One very important study showed that subjects who started their day with two or three eggs felt fuller longer and were less likely to overeat later in the day.

The Other Protein Picks

On the PrayFit Diet, you'll encounter a number of quality, high-protein food sources, and not all of them will be as obvious as beef, chicken, or fish. But just because they don't get top billing doesn't mean they're not important. While we welcome you to venture outside of the menu from time to time, it helps to know what type of breakdown you should be looking for in the foods you choose to support your weight loss. Each item in our meal plan was handpicked, not only for its protein content but for the other factors that it brings to the table. Here are some of the protein-heavy foods that help to speed and sustain results.

Food	Serving Size	Protein (g)	X Factors
Egg white	1 large	4	Contains less saturated fat than whole eggs
Ezekiel tortilla	1 tortilla	6	High in fiber; complete protein source
Almond butter	1 tablespoon	2	Tastes fantastic; very portable
Hard-boiled egg	1 large	6	Easy way to get quality protein on the go
Black beans, cooked	1 cup	15	High fiber content further slows digestion
Cottage cheese	4 ounces	14	Also has muscle- and bone-friendly calcium
String cheese	1 piece	6	Can be had anywhere; variety of types
Ground turkey	4 ounces	22	Lighter way to enjoy burgers; offers many seasoning options
Greek yogurt	⅔ cup	11	More protein, less sugar than regular yogurt
Pork chops	1 chop	33	Big on taste, shorter on calories than beef
Almonds	1 ounce	6	Heavy on healthy fats in addition to protein
Shrimp	3 ounces	18	All the benefits of fish fats in bite-sized doses

FISH PROTEIN. Fish, when prepared well, can provide great variety in a well-balanced diet, especially if you are accustomed to a lot of beef and poultry. The oils from fish are also great for reducing inflammation, protecting your heart, and shedding unwanted body fat. One study shows that subjects who consumed supplemental fish oil were able to add muscle and lose fat over a six-week period because these oils impede a stress hormone called cortisol, which can quickly break muscle down. In other words, fish lets more protein get where it needs to! In the next chapter you'll learn much more about the benefits of fish in your diet, but for the purposes of this chapter we'll focus on one: it is one of the best protein sources you can eat.

Fish is loaded with muscle-fortifying protein. Anecdotally, fish tends to help you build and hold on to muscle without causing any kind of unwanted bloating or swelling, as can sometimes be the case with fatty cuts of beef. Fish is also practically devoid of carbohydrates, leaving you room to get that fuel elsewhere, be it a healthy salad or a side dish of whole-wheat pasta. Peripherally, the healthy fats from fish oil have been shown to increase protein synthesis, the process by which muscle is built.

On the PrayFit Diet, you'll encounter savory recipes for tuna, tilapia, and salmon but there are plenty of healthy choices you can make in the fish department to bolster your protein intake.

Fish	Protein (grams) per 3-ounce serving
Salmon	23
Tuna, steak	25
Tuna, canned	22
Tilapia	21
Cod	20
Swordfish	22
Rainbow trout	21
Halibut	23
Sole	21

PROTEIN FOR VEGETARIANS. Yes, it's true: animal sources of protein such as poultry, beef, and fish are the backbone of the PrayFit

Diet. But they're not the only sources. Vegetarians can also work toward a higher daily caloric intake from protein by focusing on these foods:

Food	Protein (grams)
Quinoa, 1 cup cooked	18
Lentils, 1 cup cooked	18
Tempeh, 100 grams	18
Black beans, 1 cup cooked	15
Kidney beans, 1 cup canned	13.4
Tofu, 4 ounces	11
Soy milk, 1 cup	7
Peanut butter, 2 tablespoons	8

2,672	Average caloric intake for men
15.6	Average percentage of daily calories from protein for men
1,803	Average caloric intake for women
15.9	Average percentage of daily calories from protein for women
33	Recommended daily percentage of calories from protein on PrayFit Diet, an amount proven to improve muscle repair and retention and support fat loss

PROTEIN: THE KING OF MACRONUTRIENTS

As we've discussed at length, of all of the macronutrients protein is arguably the most underrated in terms of its potential effect on your health and body composition. Protein is in every cell, tissue, and organ in the body, meaning that you can't skimp on it. Everything from your heart to your hair and all the way down to the cross-shaped proteins called laminins that bind your cells together is made up of this crucial macronutrient.

On the PrayFit Diet, you'll get a third of your daily calories from quality, body-beneficial protein. At 4 calories per gram, that means you'll take in about 600 calories, or about 150 grams of clean, lean protein per day. You will achieve this by eating some amount of protein at every meal. How do you reach 150 grams of protein? If your day includes 4 egg whites, a cup of Greek yogurt, 6 ounces of roasted or grilled chicken breast, 2 tablespoons of peanut butter, and 6 ounces of cooked salmon, for example, you're there! The meal plans beginning on page 127 will illustrate even more specifics.

Getting this quantity of healthy protein will help you to maximize muscle repair and retention, decrease overeating, support your workouts, and speed your weight loss.

PrayFit's recipe-designer extraordinaire Dana White knows a thing or two about developing easy-to-remember guidelines for clients and readers. "Remember, a 3-ounce portion of protein is about the size of an iPhone," she says. "Here are some other easy protein gram counts to remember."

Food	Protein Count (in grams)
Grilled chicken breast, 3 ounces	25
Greek yogurt, 1 cup	13
Milk, 1 cup	11
Cooked beans, ½ cup	8
Almonds, ¼ cup	8
Peanut butter, 2 tablespoons	7

TURN YOUR TABLES

My wife is the runner in the family, and I typically don't read her magazine, but the cover blurb on an old *Runner's World* caught my eye: "The Most Inspiring Runner You've Never Met." And I can tell you that if he's not, he's close.

Hit by a car at the age of six, Bret Dunlap spent weeks in a coma. His first word when he woke up? "No." Seems he knew he had more life in him. And while he doesn't remember saying that, the life he lived for the thirty-nine years after the accident simply prove that he sure meant it. And something his mom said to him stuck with me. She said, "God never said anything about fair. He said you got a chance." This she said to a boy who suffered brain damage and paralysis, who had a colostomy, whose face freezes, and whose mind forgets what he learns—just to name a few of his afflictions. But this she also said to a boy who would teach himself several languages, give twelve gallons of blood over the years as a volunteer, play the piano left-handed, hold the same job for over eighteen years, and eventually run. Oh, my friends, he may finish last, but he runs his race, one floppy foot after another.

Have you ever wallowed? Ever thought, "Why me?" or stomped your feet and said, "Not fair!"? I know I have. I know I *do*. But it's stories like Bret's that help give me perspective. And hope. And courage. And it's stories like Bret's that always seem to remind me of grace and what Jesus did for me on the cross. That's the honest truth of why we need to make better choices at the table. God's grace really is all I need and want, so whatever else I have in life is a gift. And when the enemy tries to convince me otherwise, when he tries to blind me to blessings, when he tries to discourage my personal calling, when he reminds me that my body is failing, I won't let it steal my joy. I'll just steal a line from Bret and say, "No."

What about you? What is *your* answer today? You know, like I said at the start of the discussion on protein, Jesus overturned tables because the temple was being mistreated, and the fact that you're reading this sentence is ironclad proof that you're ready to treat the temple—your body—with better care and concern.

Indeed, you're ready to overturn your table. You're ready to begin choosing the right kinds and amounts of protein to ignite your metabolism, build lean tissue, and support a healthy immune system. The fact that you know now just exactly the purpose of protein, its sources, and its benefits is enough to make you see the plate on your table completely differently—overturning tables when the temple is mistreated. It's our legacy as believers. Read on and continue to arm yourself with the know-how to do precisely that.

KEY PROTEIN TAKEAWAYS

† Inadequate protein consumption can be dangerous.

† Muscle is metabolic tissue that constantly consumes calories, even at rest.

† Increasing protein consumption decreases overeating by promoting fullness.

† Lean protein sources are readily used by the body to repair muscle and support fat loss.

† Eating protein at every meal keeps your body's metabolic furnace firing while maintaining muscle mass.

5

DON'T FEAR FAT

HOW TO EAT THE RIGHT KIND OF FAT, IN THE RIGHT PROPORTIONS, TO SHED POUNDS

A silhouette appears on the horizon. It's too far away to distinguish who it is, but the father who's been waiting for his son to come home can't help but wonder. Squinting, he raises his hand over his eyes to block the sun's glare. As the distant figure gets closer, the father begins to walk in that direction, slowly at first, trying to match the pace of his visitor, until he realizes that this is no visitor. It's his boy. His long-lost son is home. And with compassion and forgiveness, he runs to him, embraces him, kisses him, clothes him, and feeds him.

You know the story. The return of the prodigal son—who squandered his prospective inheritance and his family's goodwill, only to return humbled and penitent—is nothing new to you. In fact, if you're a repeat dieter, always vowing to stick to a restrictive eating plan only to fail a few days or weeks later, you may feel like you're living the tale, stuck in a loop of good intentions followed by failure and remorse. You're not squandering your inheritance, but perhaps you feel the burden of squandering away your inherited *health*.

It's not like you set out to eat poorly. But long hours at work, unrelenting obligations, deadlines, family matters, friends that matter, must-see TV, and your must-read social media all conspire to pull you off course. Before you know it, you're on foreign soil, far from your healthy intentions, in a place where you (and your body) were never designed to be. Maybe it's time to go home.

Healthy habits *shouldn't* be foreign to us—they're the way God intended for us to live. But many forces have conspired to obscure this truth. There was a time when low-fat diets were the first, best solution offered by doctors for those who had gained a few too many inches around the waist or a few too many pounds on the scale. The wisdom is hard to argue: since fat is so much more calorically dense than carbs or protein, you stand to drop plenty of weight by simply lowering fat intake. And in a "calories in, calories out" kind of world, where experts tell you to simply burn more energy than you take in as your can't-miss weight-loss strategy, fat-restricted diets are easy to understand.

Adding fuel to the fire were reports of high-fat diets being linked to heart disease and other obesity-related illnesses. Fat on your dinner plate, the thinking went, meant fat on your body.

However, time and research have caught up to the war on dietary fat, and the headlines now paint a vastly different portrait of this maligned macronutrient. Consuming more healthy dietary fat, as it turns out, is beneficial for overall health and weight loss.

As with the other macronutrients, however, balance and selection play a huge role in determining just how much fat can help you. Going too low with your daily consumption denies you the benefits it can provide to your heart, joints, and body composition. Going too high will surely lead to fat retention and other peripheral maladies. And bad choices can spell dietary doom as well. Deep-fried, oily indulgences remain on your physician's no-fly list, and for good reason. Too much of a bad thing will yield bad results. Ezekiel discusses how a vine planted in good soil near abundant water grew to be a "splendid vine" (Ezekiel 17:8). Scarfing down a plateful of bacon-wrapped corn dogs in the name of reaching your fat quota for the day is akin to planting your vine in Crisco.

Luckily, getting a grasp on a proper relationship with dietary fat is easier than you may think. The trick is to learn the difference between good and bad fats and how they affect your body, and then learn how to incorporate the good ones into your day.

You might think that a diet that calls for 33 percent of your daily calories from fat—as we do here—seems like a bad idea. But it's not. On an 1,800-calorie diet, that comes out to 600 calories, or about 67 grams of fat. When healthy fat sources are eaten in balance with the other two macronutrients (carbs and protein), this quantity of fat can actually encourage fat loss, support energy levels, and boost overall health. Still skeptical? You'll be reassured when we calm the winds of misinformation in this chapter and show you how to make fat work *for* you, without ending up *on* you.

ALL FAT IS NOT CREATED EQUAL

All fats are heavy on calories, coming in at 9 calories per gram. Carbs and protein, meanwhile, contain 4 calories per gram, making fats the heavy hitter of the macronutrient family. And like the physicians of yesteryear might say, more fat equals more calories equals more body fat equals health problems. This is true—*if* you eat the wrong types of fat.

Monounsaturated fatty acids (MUFAs) and polyunsaturated fatty acids (PUFAs) are the superstars of the fat family. These are the good fats that you'll need to get to know a bit better. Saturated fats, which should be more closely monitored, and trans fats, which should be avoided, are the unhealthy fats that give them all a bad name.

Healthy Fats

Can fat actually be healthy? Absolutely. There are two types that bear closer examination here: monounsaturated and polyunsaturated. You have probably heard both types mentioned before, but if you're like most people, once you hear "fat," you probably tuned out. But monounsaturated fats can actually help to lower cholesterol levels and aid in fat loss, while certain polyunsaturated fats improve heart health, reduce the risk of some types of cancer, and aid fat burning.

Monounsaturated fats are found in foods such as olive and canola oil, avocados, peanut butter. Take in salmon, safflower oil, walnuts, and sunflower seeds and you're getting a healthy dose of polyunsaturated fats. A great many foods will contain some blend of both. All of them are good for you, so long as you don't overload and shatter your calorie ceiling for the day.

There are added bonuses for eating a balanced diet that includes these fat sources. Mono- and polyunsaturated fats help to lower total blood cholesterol and triglycerides and raise healthy HDL cholesterol levels in the blood. They can also help to prevent chronic inflammatory-related diseases such as cardiovascular disease, and research shows that they may improve insulin sensitivity and blood pressure, reducing the risk of diabetes and hypertension, as well as helping to prevent certain cancers. And while carbs are the body's preferred energy source, these fats are also readily burned for fuel to provide you with more energy throughout the day. Plus here's the kicker: research shows that the omega-3 fats can actually activate key genes that help to burn fat while turning off genes that increase fat storage. Additional studies have shown that those who increased their monounsaturated fat intake lost weight without decreasing their overall calories.

FOODS CONTAINING HEALTHY FATS

Monounsaturated Fats (Healthy)	Polyunsaturated Fats (Healthy)
Nuts	Soybean oil
Canola oil	Canola oil
Olive oil	Walnuts
High oleic safflower oil	Flaxseed
Sunflower oil	Trout
Avocado	Herring
	Salmon

Unhealthy Fats

Those donuts in the office break room and outside the sanctuary at church are loaded with trans fat. That lunch of double burger and fries you always get is full of trans fats and artery-clogging saturated fat. If you find yourself chomping down these types of foods too often, you are setting yourself up for a world of disappointment.

While you can't completely eliminate these fats from your diet—saturated fat is in many foods that are otherwise healthy—it is important to limit these types of fat to the extent that you are able.

Trans fats form when vegetable oil is hardened via a process called hydrogenation—they are essentially unsaturated fats that have been artificially saturated with hydrogen atoms. Unfortunately, this corruptive process results in a source of fat that has been shown to increase body fat gain and promote cardiovascular disease, diabetes, and certain cancers. The exact biomechanical methods that produce the health issues associated with trans fats are not fully understood, but the association between their consumption and disease cannot be denied.

Trans fat can raise LDL levels (that's the "bad" cholesterol), stressing your heart beyond measure over time. Adding to the trans fat rap sheet is the fact that it can enhance muscle breakdown, which is bad for those trying to gain strength, add muscle, or lose body fat.

Saturated fats, which are fatty acids that are naturally saturated with hydrogen, are like the good kid that fell in with a bad crowd. While this type of fat is associated with a higher risk of cardiovascular disease, there are studies that show diets moderate in fat (around 30 percent of calories) in which 10 percent of the fat is saturated did not carry an increased risk of mortality. Saturated fats, in moderation, can actually positively impact strength levels and other hormones that influence fat loss and muscle retention. You can get a bit of this in your diet through red meat, pork, dark-meat chicken, whole milk, cheese, and butter, but don't overdo it—keep your intake of saturated fat under 20 percent of overall fat each day. You can also keep this quota in line by choosing leaner, less marbled cuts of meat such as round and sirloin, trimming visible fat off your meats, removing the skin from poultry, skimming the fat from soups and stews by chilling

FOODS WITH UNHEALTHY FATS

Saturated Fats (Eat in Moderation)	Trans Fats (Avoid)
High-fat cheeses	Margarine, hydrogenated shortening
High-fat cuts of meat	Fried foods
Whole milk, cream	Commercial pastries, cookies, crackers
Full-fat ice cream	Chips
Palm oil	Biscuits
Coconut oil	

them and removing the fat that hardens at the top, using lower-fat spreads made with healthy fats instead of butter, and choosing skim milk over higher-fat versions.

Fat Truth

So in a nutshell—a nutshell that likely once contained a great source of healthy fat—eating more of the right fats can help you live longer and leaner than skipping them entirely. The PrayFit Diet derives a full 33 percent of its daily calories from fat, mostly from mono- and polyunsaturated sources such as nuts, seeds, avocados, and olive oil. A smaller portion of saturated fat will come from animal sources such as meat and dairy because they contain quality protein, calcium, and other vitamins and minerals.

Getting 33 percent of calories from fat may seem high for those wanting to shed weight, but consider the research. As I noted in Chapter 2, a study out of Loma Linda University in California concluded that a higher-fat diet consisting of 39 percent fat, mostly from the healthy sources we've outlined, and 32 percent carbohydrates resulted in a 56 percent greater fat loss that a diet composed of 53 percent carbs and only 18 percent fat. You can't get past the evidence. The proper intake of the right fats means good things for your brain and body. Just thirty-three days on the PrayFit Diet will have you convinced not only that low-fat diets are a relic of a bygone era of misinformation and quick fixes, but also that a moderate amount of healthy fats actually can help you feel better than you imagined.

HOW TO EAT HEALTHY FATS
ON THE PRAYFIT DIET

Now that you know a bit more about healthy fats and the types that are most conducive to slimming your waist and keeping your heart healthy, we can get into the particulars of the sources that work best. These superfats all offer different benefits, but what they all have in common is great taste. Yes, fat tastes good—even when it's good for you.

At 9 calories per gram, that means you'll take in about 600 calories, or about 67 grams, of heart-healthy, joint-friendly fat per day. Sixty-seven grams of fat, said out loud . . . well that sounds like a lot. But we're not talking about mowing it all down in one setting, as is the case all too often in our less discriminate culture of heavy plates. To reach 67 grams over the course of a day doesn't take much—two eggs, a third of a cup of almonds, a tablespoon of olive oil, and a 6-ounce helping of salmon gets you there in a way that is easy, efficient, and *good for you*. The meal plans beginning on page 125 illustrate even more healthy ways to reach your fat quota for each day.

Fish

Despite being a powerful protein, fish usually takes a backseat to chicken and beef in most diets. This is unfortunate, as many types of fish are rich in omega-3 fatty acids—essential fats that the body cannot produce on its own. The two main types of omega-3s—eicosapentaenoic acid (EPA) and docosahexaenoic acid (DHA)—help to reduce inflammatory hormones and cut the risk of heart disease, diabetes, and cancer. Omega-3s improve joint health, which is great for those who work out hard or whose joints are starting to disagree with them more often than not. And think about this: they enhance brain function, too. And both EPA and DHA help to crank up your body's fat-fighting furnace and overall metabolism while also increasing protein synthesis, or muscle repair.

On the practical side, a well-prepared fish meal also offers a nice respite from the usual array of healthy foods found in diet books. Salmon has the highest content of omega-3s but other swimmers like sardine, mackerel, and tuna are all solid picks when you need to vary your protein sources. Several of these gilled delicacies appear in the PrayFit Diet but can be switched almost interchangeably without throwing off your macronutrient balance.

If you're not too keen on fish, you can still get your EPA and DHA supplementally through fish oil, aiming for 1 to 2 grams three times daily with food.

Salmon, 3 ounces | Calories: 175 | Fat: 10 grams | Saturated fat:
2 grams

Tuna, canned, 3 ounces | Calories: 99 | Fat: 1 gram | Saturated fat:
0 grams

THE OMEGA OPTIONS

In these pages, we'll be providing you with a handful of healthy recipes, but it never hurts to have a few more prep options in your repertoire. Here are a few ways you can enjoy omega-3-rich salmon.

† **SMOKED:** Prepared smoked salmon is a great alternative when you don't have time to cook. Wrap it around asparagus stalks for a fancy but effortless appetizer or along with a salad for a light meal.

† **POACHED:** Cooking salmon in a bath of wine, water, and spices infuses it with flavor while keeping it tender and flaky without drastically affecting calorie count.

† **GRILLED:** Thread chunks of skinless salmon onto skewers and grill for dinner in minutes. Sprinkle it with a spice rub to add big flavor without marinating.

† **WRAPPED:** Wrap salmon fillets in foil packets with lemon and fresh herbs for quick cooking and easy cleanup.

† **SEARED:** For a tasty burger, finely chop fresh salmon in the food processor, flavor it up with sweet pineapple and spicy chili pepper, then give it a quick sear in a nonstick skillet.

When you visit the fish counter in search of quality salmon, you're most likely going to run into Atlantic salmon. In general, this is an affordable and healthy salmon, so you can be confident that you're getting your healthy-fat fix when you lay down the bucks for it. But when you get your pick of fillets, always go with the thicker cut. Taken from the center of the fish, rather than near the well-muscled tail, this cut will be more tender and rich. For the uninitiated, fresh salmon will be bright orange in color and doesn't smell very "fishy." If your cut is off-color, slimy, or particularly fragrant, find a new place to buy it.

Avocado

A good, perfectly ripe avocado is a great thing to have in your countertop fruit bowl. It is tasty and colorful, and it packs a wallop in the healthy fats category. A medium avocado, which is roughly 5 ounces, has 226 calories, 3 grams of protein, and—wait for it—9 grams of fiber. See Chapter 3 to find out why that last stat alone is enough to start loving avocado. But since our focus here is fat, this is the grabber: 80 percent of that avocado's calories come from heart-healthy monounsaturated fats.

The fat from avocados has been shown to defend against cancer, offset visible signs of aging, and elevate natural growth hormone production, which is imperative for maximizing fat burning. And unlike the fat you'd get from a meal heavier in saturated or trans fat, the fat from avocados won't slow you down. In fact, monounsaturated fat is easily burned for fuel during activity.

Avocados are also off-the-charts high in potassium and are replete with calcium and magnesium, all of which are important for helping you maintain high levels of muscle function and fluid balance during activity. Plus avocados contain mannoheptulose, a sugar that actually blunts insulin release, helping to discourage fat retention.

Use avocados in a salad, in sandwiches and wraps, or as part of a tasty guacamole dip—the kitchen options for this healthy, fat-laden fruit are virtually unlimited.

Avocado, 1 ounce | Calories: 47 | Fat: 4 grams | Saturated fat: 1 gram

Olive Oil

If fats on the whole have been demonized by the media over the years, it would seem that olive oil has contracted a separate public relations agency. This seemingly ubiquitous superfat has become to cooking what my Yankees are to baseball: a timeless partnership. Olive oil as an industry has flourished in recent years, with the United States importing fifty million gallons per year. That's a lot of fat flooding the market, sure, but this is one that you shouldn't be without. The fat from olive oil helps to lower bad cholesterol, fights high blood pressure, and keeps your arteries clean and clear. Olive oil is also used by many as a digestive aid.

Rich in monounsaturated fats—1 tablespoon contains 10 grams of it—olive oil has tons of uses. You're not likely to be left scratching your head at a way to build it into your diet.

Again, in modest helpings, olive oil can be used as a butter substitute or a cooking aid (choose pure olive oil for this). Virgin and extra-virgin varieties are terrific drizzled over salads.

Olive oil, 1 tablespoon | Calories: 114 | Fat: 14 grams | Saturated fat: 2 grams

Peanut Butter

To this day, peanut butter is one of my favorite foods. (I grew up eating peanut butter and honey sandwiches; how about a show of hands from those who join me in such amazing praise of them?) Indeed, from our brown-bag lunches in the schoolyard to sneaked spoonfuls just before bedtime, there's something special about our relationship with peanut butter. Each decadent, creamy spoonful is more than just a treat—it's an experience. Still, most people don't realize that every time they consume one of America's favorite foods, they're ingesting a powerful dose of health. Not only is your PB rich in protein, but it is loaded with monounsaturated fat. One tablespoon contains 4 grams of protein and 8 grams of fat. It's also a moderate-carb snack if you keep it in check, at 6 grams per tablespoon.

But when purchasing your peanut butter, be particular. You'll want to select a jar that has little more than peanuts and salt as its main ingredients. This will help to ensure that you're not inadvertently eating hidden sugars or unhealthy trans fats.

One of the ideal times to nosh on peanut butter is just before bedtime. Because it is a solid combination of protein and fat, it slows digestion down to a crawl while you sleep, which is ideal for preserving muscle and maximizing recovery from activity or exercise.

You can have it by itself, from the spoon—that's the way nature intended it, right?—or in conjunction with a healthy dipping object such as celery or apple slices. Unfortunately the J to your PB isn't always a great idea—the sugar from the jelly can result in unwanted body fat. Reserve the jelly for post-workout periods when your body is less likely to store those sugars as fat.

Peanut butter, 2 tablespoons | Calories: 188 | Fat: 16 grams | Saturated fat: 3 grams

Nuts

The Lord knows your heart. And the American Heart Association knows hearts. So when the AHA says that something is good for your ticker, you had better believe it knows what it's talking about. The lab coats at the AHA recommend having a handful of nuts (about 1.5 ounces) per day. Why? Because 80 percent of the nut—and this applies to most nut varieties—consists of heart-friendly, monounsaturated fat and plenty of fiber. Nuts can lower cholesterol, reduce heart stress caused by free radicals, and decrease inflammation.

Pick your favorite, because most are good for you. Walnuts would probably sit atop the leaderboard if we were keeping score. They have been extensively studied and have been shown repeatedly to boost heart health. One recent study found that walnuts are higher in antioxidants than other nuts. Antioxidants protect cells against damage caused by harmful molecules known as free radicals, which can play a role in heart disease. Add to that the fact that walnuts have been shown to improve circulation and you have the makings of a nut dynasty. But the other nuts in the family aren't exactly slouches. You can expect similar benefits from all of them, provided that you don't douse them in salt or chocolate.

Another great thing about nuts is their portability—no microwave or cold storage required. If you have a small plastic bag, you're good to go. Not surprisingly, it's important to watch how many nuts you eat. Because they're so high in fat, and because they are such a tasty snack, it can be easy to lose track of how much you've had. A good way to measure the requisite 1.5 ounces is to pour them in your cupped palm without brimming over or dropping any. In the case of almonds, for example, this usually equates to twenty nuts or so.

Type of nut	Calories	Total fat (saturated/unsaturated fat)
Almonds, raw	163	14 g (1.1 g/12.2 g)
Almonds, dry-roasted	169	15 g (1.1 g/12.9 g)
Brazil nuts, raw	186	19 g (4.3 g/12.8 g)
Cashews, dry-roasted	163	13.1 g (2.6 g/10 g)
Chestnuts, roasted	69	0.6 g (0.1 g/0.5 g)
Hazelnuts (filberts), raw	178	17 g (1.3 g/15.2 g)
Hazelnuts (filberts), dry-roasted	183	17.7 g (1.3 g/15.6 g)
Macadamia nuts, raw	204	21.5 g (3.4 g/17.1 g)
Macadamia nuts, dry-roasted	204	21.6 g (3.4 g/17.2 g)
Peanuts, dry-roasted	166	14 g (2 g/11.4 g)
Pecans, dry-roasted	201	21 g (1.8 g/18.3 g)
Pistachios, dry-roasted	161	12.7 g (1.6 g/10.5 g)
Walnuts, halved	185	18.5 g (1.7 g/15.9 g)

Source: Mayo Clinic

HEALTHY FAT PROFILE: FLAXSEED

It can be tough working enough healthy fat into your diet. The meal plans that begin on page 125 will help you get on the right track. But for people who have been programmed to think that more dietary fat is just a quick ticket to more belly fat, it can be even more laborious. Luckily, one fantastic source of healthy fatty acids—flaxseed—can be worked into your diet in a few crafty, less obvious ways.

Flaxseed is an excellent source of alpha-lineoleic acid, which is converted to EPA and DHA in the body—the same superfats found in fish. Both flaxseeds and flaxseed oil pack a potent punch (you can also grind flaxseed if you desire). Just 1 tablespoon of flaxseeds contains 55 calories, including 4 grams of fat—all of it healthy. Here's how to get more of it into your diet to hit your 33 percent quota for healthy dietary fat calories.

† **IN A SHAKE:** You'll find a smoothie or two on the PrayFit Diet, and many of you will have your own recipes that fall within the given meal plan param-

eters. By adding a tablespoon (or two) of flaxseeds or flaxseed oil, you can add healthy fat and some welcome texture to your smoothie without really altering the flavor.

† **WITH YOUR OATS:** Many breakfasts will call for oatmeal. Sprinkle some flaxseed into the mix to punch up this already high-fiber morning favorite.

† **IN BAKING:** You can easily mix flaxseed or flaxseed oil into many of your favorite baking recipes to increase the amount of heart-healthy fat you're getting. For example, you can throw a few tablespoons of flax into a whole-grain pancake mix or into a batch of homemade bran muffins to get whole grains and healthy fats without sacrificing flavor.

We had a rule growing up: if my brother and I got in trouble for doing something wrong, we weren't allowed to keep pouting about it. Yes, we suffered consequences, but it wasn't held over our heads—once it was done, it was over, finished, like it never happened. In fact, if I was pouting about it later on, you guessed it—I got in trouble for pouting. You know what that taught me? Trust. I trusted my parents. I knew what to expect. Periodically reprimanded, constantly loved.

Although he came back with memories of deeds as stinky as his pig-slop-covered clothes, the prodigal son couldn't stray beyond his father's love. Before he knew it, a robe replaced his rags, a ring dressed his hand, and a feast filled his belly. And while you and I may not have mud on our shoes, there's not a person reading this sentence who doesn't need that kind of grace from a grace-giving God.

Plainly said, many of us have treated our bodies—our inherited health—much like the prodigal son treated the inheritance that his father gave him early. We've overspent and wasted it. But something tells me the prodigal son took better care of the things he was given after he got home. And so can we. For some, there's a family waiting for you, too—waiting for you to start eating better. They're waiting to celebrate you. Who's coming home, been home, staying home? You're the life of their party. It doesn't begin without you. Indeed, you know the story. You're writing it right now. It's your life. When the prodigal son returned, what does the Bible say the family ate in celebration? "Bring the fattened calf . . . let's have a feast and celebrate . . . for this son of mine was dead and is alive again" (Luke 15:23–24). Consider this diet your welcome-home feast. The fact that you're alive is reason to celebrate. Let's eat.

KEY FAT TAKEAWAYS

† Fats are higher in calories than carbs or protein.
† Keeping fats in balance aids heart health, joints, and weight loss.
† Healthy fats include monounsaturated and polyunsaturated fats.
† Aim for a moderate intake of saturated fat.
† Eliminate dangerous trans fats.
† Good fats are found in fish, avocado, peanut butter, and more.

PART III

THE PRAYFIT PLAN

6

BUILDING
THE PRAYFIT PLATE

I've been extremely humbled and blessed to receive a few awards throughout my life and career, but one stands out as my most cherished. When I was a kid, my coaches gave me the "Hustle Award." Ironically, it was for a sport that I wasn't particularly great at: basketball. Try to imagine someone running the 100-meter hurdles wearing swim fins. Got the visual? That's me playing hoops. And even *that* might be kind.

But while I didn't run the offense very well or lead the team in rebounds, and although I was never the game's high scorer, I was never outhustled. For whatever reason—whether it was at practice or in a game—something inside my heart just would not let me be outworked.

You know, they don't give hustle awards after you grow up. But think about it. When you're the only one in the office unwilling to gossip, that's hustle. When you get up extra early each day to make sure your kids eat a balanced breakfast, that's hustle. And when you lace up those running shoes minutes after taking off the work ones, that's hustle.

As believers, we have faith. And because of that truth, regardless of the situation, we should never be outworked. When someone wonders what makes the difference in us, why we're not like the crowd at school or at work, or why we're beginning this new balanced approach to food, it's because faith is in our hearts. Hearts that beat. Hearts that hustle.

As you build your PrayFit Plate, have that mind-set. You won't be outworked. You're hustling for better health for all the *right* reasons. And because those reasons don't fade over time, neither do you.

PUTTING YOUR BALANCED PLATE INTO ACTION

The PrayFit Diet aims to reconfigure our relationship with food— never eating for vanity or gluttony but rather taking a hard line on a perfect proportion of foods that provide exactly what our body needs. Not more, not less.

And that's the beauty of the macronutrient ratio, 33-33-33, that we advocate here. By consuming the proper carbohydrates, lean proteins, and healthy fats in equal amounts, you receive the synergistic benefits that all three have to offer. No more glazed eyes on the road through the morning commute or heavy eyes at three o'clock. No more debilitating sugar cravings midmorning and no more rummaging through the pantry just before bedtime. With the PrayFit Diet, you won't need to. By bringing your macronutrients into balance, you can experience higher levels of energy, faster weight loss, fewer cravings, a speedier metabolism, and a new perspective on what it means to be fulfilled by food.

This month-plus of education is the greatest favor you can do for the body that God so intricately crafted in His own image. And by the time it's over, your body will better reflect your gratitude for such a gift.

DAY 34: BUILD ON DAYS 1–33

One of the best ways to learn something is through repetition. And when these thirty-three days come to an end, you will have prepared more than a hundred delicious, good-for-you meals and snacks. The great thing about that is that will have ingrained in your mind what a healthy, balanced meal looks like. How does that help? You'll forgive the analogy, but people who work at the U.S. Treasury don't study counterfeit bills. They know what they look like, of course, but it's because they spend hours on end studying the *real thing*. That way, when a fake comes across their desk, they know it right away. We need to do the same thing with our plate.

In other words, learning what healthy foods and reasonable proportions look like is one of the best ways to instill these types of habits for good. You'll be better able to determine when your plate is out of balance, no matter where you are. You'll know instinctively if your plate is loaded with sources of readily available energy or foodstuffs that are merely destined to cause you harm. You'll be able to tell—without consulting a chart or calculator—whether your meal contains the balance that you now know to be ideal for reducing inflammation and promoting weight loss.

The PrayFit Diet is prescriptive, make no mistake. But that prescription is also steeped in education, which is why we've provided you everything you need to know about food to achieve your ideal body weight. We haven't weighed these pages down with unnecessary mathematics or burdensome, militant menus. We've simply issued a call for a return to the basics—eating what we need to fulfill our purpose here on earth.

To reinforce these broader guidelines, we'll take a final look at how your ideal day should shape up. We'll describe what types of foods are optimal for certain times of the day and provide some quick examples of what those foods would be. You are welcome to consult the detailed menus later in the book for even more precise suggestions for your thirty-three days of meals.

IDENTIFYING THE REAL DEAL

Once you know what a genuinely balanced, healthy meal looks like, you'll be able to sniff out an impostor with relatively little effort. This table pits meal against meal, snack against snack. Think you can spot the fake? Give it a go, then see what our resident nutritionist has to say about your guess.

Breakfast 1	Breakfast 2
1 bowl of oatmeal with cinnamon sugar	2 eggs
1 cup orange juice	1 whole-wheat English muffin
1 cup coffee	1 tablespoon natural peanut butter
	1 banana
	Water
Winner	

Breakfast 2

WHY? Breakfast 1, which many people might think is a strong choice, has too much added sugar and carbs. Also, there's not a good source of protein in sight! Breakfast 2 has a clear balance of nutrients—protein and healthy fats in the eggs and peanut butter, whole-grain, slowly digested carbs in the English muffin for lasting energy, and a serving of fruit. This is a much more nutrient-dense meal!

Lunch 1	Lunch 2
5 ounces grilled chicken breast	Chicken breast sandwich with
½ cup cooked brown rice	BBQ sauce
½ cup cooked black beans	Veggie chips
¼ cup salsa	Diet soda
Water	
Winner	

Lunch 1

WHY? Lunch 1 is the clear winner here. This is a hunger-fighting meal, packed with fiber and protein to give you lasting energy. Salsa, which is filled with vitamins and minerals, is a much better condiment choice than sugary BBQ sauce. And there are studies that show that those who consume diet soda may be at greater risk for weight gain because, as in this example, they tend to overdo it with other poor food choices.

Dinner 1	Dinner 2
Regular spaghetti with beef	2 cups cooked spaghetti squash
meat sauce	with turkey meat sauce
2 breadsticks	2 cups baby spinach
Caesar salad	1 tablespoon olive oil + balsamic
Diet soda	vinegar
	Water
Winner	

Dinner 2

WHY? Dinner 2 wins here, hands down. This dinner is made with turkey meat sauce, giving it a lower-fat, higher-protein punch. And instead of traditional pasta, it uses spaghetti squash—a veggie instead of a rapidly digested carb. Also, olive oil and balsamic vinegar are a much lighter choice than Caesar dressing. Again, the diet soda doesn't make up for the rest of the dinner. Water would be a better choice.

(continued on next page)

Snack 1	Snack 2
¼ cup almonds	1 apple
1 hard-boiled egg	6 ounces pretzels
Winner	
Snack 1	

WHY? Snack 1 is simply a much higher-quality snack—no processed ingredients or added sugar, just pure protein and healthy fats. Some people may be quick to reach for the pretzels because they're convenient, but you can prepare hard-boiled eggs in bulk and keep almonds handy in your car or office, so you can always have something much more filling and balanced to get you through to your next meal.

BREAKFAST

Your parents were telling you the truth, of course. Breakfast really is the most important meal of the day. It is here, at this meal, that you lay the foundation for a day of healthy eating. Skip it, wait too long to eat it, or make the wrong choices, and all of the hours that follow are likely to be bound in nutritional sorrows and misery. Missteps during this crucial window interrupt your nutritional flow, so to speak, and can have a detrimental effect on weight-loss goals.

Don't Skip It

If you think that rushing out the door without having breakfast is going to save you calories and help you lose weight, think again. Researchers at Cornell University found that people who skip breakfast tend to crave more carbohydrates later in the day compared with test subjects who eat breakfast. So while you may want to pat yourself on the back for skipping your usual bagel and cream cheese first thing in the morning, you're likely to have two or three of them later. Another study from the Dairy Research Institute found that people who skip breakfast weigh more and have more unhealthy habits than those who eat breakfast. Those who skip breakfast also consume 40 percent more sweets, 55 percent more soft drinks, 45 percent fewer vegetables, and 30 percent less fruit than people who eat breakfast.

Need more incentive? A new study from the Sussex Innovation Centre in Brighton, United Kingdom, found that eating breakfast improves people's mental performance. Over 60 percent of test subjects showed improvements in English and mathematics tests after eating breakfast. Hand-eye coordination was also improved. Furthermore, breakfast eaters showed a reduction in anxiety levels when faced with stressful situations.

> 44: Percentage of Americans who skip breakfast on a daily basis.

Don't Wait

Other than after a workout, there is no time of day when your body is more starved for nutrients than first thing in the morning. Just because you're sleeping doesn't mean that your body has stopped burning fuel. In fact, your brain runs all night on fuel from stored sugars, or glycogen, and when that stock is exhausted, it starts converting your muscles' amino acids into glucose for fuel. That's not a good thing, since holding on to muscle is crucial for supporting weight loss. The longer you go without replenishing your body's fuel stores, the more you are at risk of compromising any progress you have made. Plus, breakfast is the best way to jump-start your mind and metabolism. A hungry brain is a sluggish brain. And your body can't start burning fuel until you've thrown some onto the fire.

Choose Wisely

The aforementioned bagel may seem like a great idea, but it is loaded with quickly digested simple sugars that cause your blood sugar first to spike and then to plummet, leaving you feeling sluggish and making you more likely to crave something else unhealthy. The same is true for many breakfast cereals, donuts, white toast, and so on—they leave your body convinced that it needs to refuel again to compensate for the drop. In desperation, you are far more likely in these circumstances to reach for something that will quickly restore blood sugar levels to normal, such as candy or other sweets. The worst part of the blood sugar roller coaster is that during lows, your body releases more insulin, a hormone that convinces your body to store fat for later. You can see how this can be a vicious cycle.

PrayFit Diet Breakfast Carbs

A better bet is to choose foods that will be digested more slowly, preventing maniacal swings in blood sugar and hormones. This is where complex carbohydrates come in. These foods, typically higher in fiber and of generally greater nutritive value, tend to serve that need well. Not only do they top off your energy stores after your slumber, but they place valuable octane in the tank for the day ahead while also staving off diet-wrecking cravings by stabilizing blood sugar.

If you're stumped about what healthy carbs to eat first thing in the morning, pick one of the foods from this tasty list—any one of them will satisfy your PrayFit serving of healthy breakfast carbs.

Rolled oats: 1 cup cooked

Ezekiel bread, tortillas: 1 piece

Whole-wheat bread: 1 slice

Whole-wheat English muffins: 1 piece

Oranges: 1 medium

Grapefruit: 1 medium

Whole-grain cereal: 1–2 cups

Berries: 1 cup

Banana: 1 medium

PrayFit Diet Breakfast Protein

Of equal importance at breakfast is the quick introduction of protein. Remember, the longer it takes for you to replenish spent energy, the more your muscles are at risk of being cannibalized by your body to fill that need, so eating adequate protein as soon as possible is paramount. But this also serves another purpose, and that's to fill you up right. You see, while quickly digested carbs will leave you sluggish and dazed, the wrong protein choice can end up making you feel heavy, slow, or even bloated. Great pains should be taken to avoid processed breakfast meats such as bacon, sausage, and chorizo. Loaded with fat and sodium, these foods can crush your productivity before you have your shoes on. Instead, shift your emphasis to proven, reliable sources of protein that halt muscle wasting and offer satiety.

If you're looking for the best types of nourishing protein to eat first thing in the morning, pick one of the foods from this list—any one of them will satisfy your PrayFit serving of healthy breakfast protein.

Eggs: 1 large egg

Egg whites: 3 large

Greek yogurt: 6–8 ounces

Peanut butter: 1–2 tablespoons

Almond butter: 1–2 tablespoons

Ezekiel bread, tortillas: 1 piece

Milk: 1 cup

Soy milk: 1 cup

PrayFit Diet Breakfast Fats

Fats also play a vital role in how your day is likely to play out. Healthy fats tend to aid in digestion and, because they are more calorie-dense, also add to your feeling of fullness. Omega-3s boost cognitive function as well.

If you're unsure about how to fit good fats into your breakfast, pick one of the foods from this tasty list—any one of them will satisfy your PrayFit serving of healthy breakfast fat.

Peanut butter: 1–2 tablespoons
Almond butter: 1–2 tablespoons
Eggs: 1 large
Granola: ¼–½ cup
Flaxseed: 1–2 tablespoons

LUNCH

One meal sets the stage for the next. So if you've fumbled your breakfast, chances are you'll fumble your lunch. Keeping your nutritional goals in mind, and thinking ahead to the next meal, it's important to refuel properly at this midday juncture.

Lunch Is a Bridge

In the awkward space between your morning eggs and your evening salmon lies lunch. Don't spoil those healthy bookends with a greasy lunch-truck burrito, a full basket of fries, or a dressed-to-the-nines chili dog. Choosing healthy fare at this time is just as healthy as it is during other times of the day—consistency breeds consistency. And when you make questionable choices during this window, you are less likely to have a healthy dinner and far less likely to keep your weight loss on track.

But also consider that when you hit midday, you have most of your day left to conquer. Providing your body with the right type and amount of food can help you avoid the 3:00 p.m. malaise that hits so many people. This is almost always due to improper lunch choices that have thrown blood sugar out of whack and expose deficiencies in other parts of self-care, such as sleep and hydration.

And since you will have likely burned through most of your breakfast, getting this meal in is important for avoiding additional dips in energy or productivity.

Lunch Is Fuel

Hopefully you have chosen to implement some type of exercise as part of your overall weight-loss strategy. And because so many of us work or go to school or care for our families during the day, that means that workouts are relegated to the evenings. As you look ahead to those workouts, it's important to continue throwing the proper kindling on the fire.

But even if you're not hitting the gym or putting on your PrayFit DVD after you punch out today, you still need to work toward your daily energy requirements and macronutrient ratios. This means that you will need to apply the same principles of balance to this meal that you did to your breakfast.

PrayFit Diet Lunch Carbs

As with breakfast, you'll need more carbs that can provide sustained energy and waist-whittling fiber. If you need suggestions for which healthy carbs to eat for lunch, look at the foods from this tasty list—any one of them will fulfill your PrayFit serving of healthy lunch carbs.

Brown rice: 1 cup cooked
Black beans: ½ cup cooked
Mixed greens: 3 cups
Spinach: 1–3 cups

Pomegranate: 1 medium

Ezekiel bread, tortillas: 1 piece

Whole-wheat pizza: 1 slice

Broccoli: 1 cup

White beans: ¼–½ cup cooked

Sweet potato: 1 medium

PrayFit Diet Lunch Protein

You also can't ignore the importance of protein. Since muscle is metabolic tissue, consuming some amount of protein every time you put fork to mouth is a great dietary default strategy. Making sure you get a lean, light source of protein at lunch helps to fill you up and provide your muscles with the amino acids they need to continue rebuilding and reshaping themselves, which contributes to greater overall fat loss. If you're unsure about what healthy protein to eat first at midday, pick one of the foods from this list—any one of them will satisfy your PrayFit serving of healthy lunch protein.

Chicken breast: 3–6 ounces

Deli turkey: 2–3 ounces

Hard-boiled egg: 1 large

Tuna: 3 ounces

Turkey breast: 3–6 ounces

Black beans: ¼–½ cup cooked

Salmon: 3–6 ounces

PrayFit Diet Lunch Fats

Again, healthy dietary fat is critical for your overall health, as well as your fat-loss efforts. The bonus here is that as satiety from breakfast subsides, these healthy fats add calories and taste while also reducing body inflammation and switching on key genes that influence fat loss. If you're stumped by what healthy fats to eat for lunch, select one of the foods from this list—any one of them will achieve your PrayFit serving of healthy lunch fat.

Cheese: 1 ounce

Fish (tuna, salmon): 3–6 ounces

Olive oil: 1 tablespoon

Peanut butter: 1–2 tablespoons

Nuts: ¼ cup

SNACKS

One of the cornerstones of the PrayFit Diet is metabolism. And by eating more often in smaller portions, you can dramatically accelerate your metabolism, the rate at which your body burns through energy. The higher your metabolism, the sleeker your physique.

That's why we add a healthy snack into each day. Ideally, this snack should come between lunch and dinner, but it can also be moved to the space between breakfast and lunch. This will force your metabolism to ramp up.

But you'll have to rethink what you know about snacks. The term "snack" is too closely associated with things such as chips, popcorn, candy, and other empty-calorie foods. In the PrayFit Diet vernacular, "snack" means sustenance. It means high-power fuel for whatever comes next. It means feeding your body, further suppressing cravings, and continuing to eat your way slimmer.

PrayFit Diet Snack Carbs

Snacks need to have a balance of macronutrients. This is, as with complete meals, designed to promote fullness, deepen energy reserves, and provide caloric adequacy. Slower-burning, fiber-rich carbs are always a great snack choice.

Baby carrots: 1 cup

Banana: 1 medium

Apple: 1 medium

Cucumber: 1 cup

Clementine: 1 medium

Orange: 1 medium

Grapefruit: 1 medium

Dried cranberries: ¼ cup

PrayFit Diet Snack Proteins

Protein also needs to be factored in. This fourth feeding should be viewed as an opportunity to fortify muscles with a quick hit of amino acids. Luckily, protein is easier to find in the snack arena than you may think. Contrary to what you might think, you don't need to roast a salmon steak in order to power up with this macronutrient.

Cottage cheese: ½–1 cup

String cheese: 1 ounce

Cheese, sliced: 1 ounce

Almonds: ¼ cup

Edamame: ½ cup

Deli turkey: 2–3 ounces

Almond butter: 1–2 tablespoons

Greek yogurt: 1 cup

PrayFit Diet Snack Fats

Remember, your snack should allow you to continue reaping the benefits that healthy dietary fat has to offer. The presence of fat in your snack also ensures that you are getting enough of the right calories at the right times. The type of fat emphasized in the PrayFit Diet won't sink you—these healthy fats can knock down appetite without knocking out your energy levels.

String cheese: 1 ounce

Cottage cheese: ½ cup

Almonds: ¼ cup

Almond butter: 1–2 tablespoons

Walnuts: ¼ cup

Hard-boiled egg: 1 large

DINNER

Dinner is a vitally important meal because you are about to rest your body. The time between your evening spread and your alarm going off can be ten hours or more for some people, meaning that your body will need enough stored energy to function well throughout the night. Also, as you close your day, your body is likely starving for fuel—this is true whether you hit the gym today or stayed at the office. Every waking moment of the day, you are consuming your body's available energy, and it needs to be replenished. And unless you are working a night shift, at dinner you may have more time to experiment with tasty recipes than in the morning.

Dinner for Refueling

Everyone's activity level and metabolism are different. That means that everyone is burning calories throughout the day to different degrees. Some will burn more, some will burn less, but by dinner, we all will have worked ourselves through the day one calorie at a time. Dinner is an opportunity to provide protein to broken-down muscles, healthy fats to aching joints, and complex carbs to start replenishing stored glycogen for the next day. This is even more important if you have worked out later in the day— say, after work but before dinner. As training exhausts stored sugars and breaks down muscle fiber, this meal may end up having the most impact on your overall fat loss.

Dinner as Insurance

As one meal builds toward the next, one day sets the stage for the next. Inadequate dinners put you at risk of greater muscle wasting as you sleep and lower starting energy levels the next morning. It also compromises tomorrow's workout by leaving you ill-equipped to improve upon today's performance in the gym. It's hard enough getting all the fuel you need while you're awake. Setting yourself up for continued success while you sleep depends largely on how good of a dinner you eat. Oh, and a balanced dinner filled with healthy protein, carbs, and fat also makes you far less likely to ransack the kitchen cabinets come nine o'clock.

Operation "Dinner In"

Eating dinner at home is always preferable to eating dinner out because you are able to control your macronutrient intake down to the gram. And because this is your last meal of the day, you want to make sure that it features a good balance of the major macronutrients.

PrayFit Diet Dinner Protein

Most dinner planning revolves around your choice of protein. Whether it's chicken, fish, beef, or pork, this is the glue that holds the rest of the plate together. Just a few ounces of clean protein can provide all the building blocks you need to keep your metabolic motor running. Protein will start the rebuilding process on weakened muscle tissue and release hormones that make you feel fuller longer. You just want to make sure that you pick the leanest types of meat available. Fatty fish, which are rich in healthy omega-3 fats, are the exception to this rule.

Chicken breast: 3–6 ounces
Fish (salmon, tuna, tilapia): 3–6 ounces (tilapia is not high in omega-3, salmon and tuna are)

Flank steak: 3–6 ounces

Ground turkey: 3–6 ounces

Chicken thighs: 3–6 ounces

Pork chops: 3–6 ounces

Pork tenderloin: 3–6 ounces

PrayFit Diet Dinner Carbs

Even though the "meat-and-potato dinner" is thought to be a quintessentially American concept, it turns out that spuds are not always the proper choice for dinner. Some healthy carbs are necessary, but complex carbs are always a better choice. Instead of the white potato, you'll go with a sweet potato. Instead of white rice, you'll try brown. Whole-wheat pastas will replace traditional noodles. Carbs aren't the enemy, not even at dinnertime. Make the right choices and you'll be set.

Whole-wheat pasta: 1–2 cups cooked

Sweet potato: 1 medium

Brown rice: 1 cup cooked

Ezekiel bread, tortillas: 1 piece

Whole-wheat crackers: 6–8 crackers

Mixed veggies: 1 cup

PrayFit Diet Dinner Fats

Fat at dinnertime? You betcha. Generous helpings of unsaturated fats and even measured portions of saturated fats are all good for continued progress on the weight-loss front. One great, easy way to get your healthy fats at dinner is by way of olive-oil-based dressings. Cheeses are also a hit at dinnertime, giving you saturated fats, along with additional protein. Keeping in mind that while some dinners will have less fat than others, as a rule you shouldn't aim to keep fats too low at dinnertime, especially since these aid in the satiety that keeps you out of the kitchen at night.

Olive oil: 1 tablespoon

Feta cheese: ¼ cup

BUILDING YOUR OWN PRAYFIT PLATE

You may be tired of hearing it by now, but it bears repeating: by eating in perfect balance among the three major macronutrients, you can lose weight, increase energy, and dramatically improve your overall health and vitality. To enjoy these benefits, you simply eat an equal amount of calories—about 600—from protein, carbs, and fat each day. With protein and carbs weighing in at 4 calories per gram and fat at 9 calories per gram, that means you get 150 grams of protein, 150 grams of carbs, and 67 grams of fat per day, every day. If you keep to these prescribed guidelines, a healthier you is just thirty-three days away.

Remember, these parameters will work for anyone between 130 and 250 pounds, but if you are slightly heavier or lighter than that, you can adjust. If you're heavier, you can allow yourself an extra 500 calories per day, and if you're lighter and find eating this many calories difficult, you can reduce your calories a bit, being careful not to fall below 1,200 per day. In both cases, the only requirement is that you keep the macronutrients balanced: 33 percent of your day's calories from each.

The meal plans that follow are written as a teaching tool—by going through the work of preparing balanced, healthy meals for thirty-three days, you'll instinctively be able to do so for the long haul. Consider it a jump start into a life of abundant living, where we've eliminated all the guesswork! You're holding the most balanced food plan and lifestyle ever designed; glory, finally.

But the next thirty-three days also serve as a test. Although the bodily and spiritual payoff is ample, we're under no illusions that this transition won't be a challenge for folks. That's why we made it thirty-three days—because not only is a month scientifically proven to be ample time to firmly establish healthy habits and lose weight, but it serves as a reminder of the reason you're doing it all in the first place. Jesus was thirty-three when He went to the cross for our sins. He gave us thirty-three years and Heaven. Let's give Him thirty-three days of faithful, mindful eating for the rest of our lives.

In the next chapters, you're going to have everything you need to get started—shopping lists, meal plans, and tasty recipes. But first, we've got to clean out your kitchen. It's time to purge your fridge and pantry of all of the foodstuffs that are weighing you down. After all, remember what Paul said: everything is permissible, but not all things are beneficial (1 Corinthians 10:23).

PANTRY CLEANSE

Now that you know everything you ever wanted to know about protein, fat, and carbs and how they work together in your body to create the ideal environment for weight loss and abundant general health, it's time to take a look at the specifics of our thirty-three-day plan.

We've discussed the nutritional and caloric parameters you'll be following during your first thirty-three days on the PrayFit Diet, and some guidelines explaining how to actually build that PrayFit Plate for breakfast, lunch, dinner, and even snacks. Now I'm about to give you some specific suggestions for how to shop with the 33 percent caloric balance in mind (and, just as important, what foods to avoid). The pages that follow will provide a vast array of foods for you to choose from, each with its own proven ability to exact positive change within the body—some because of how they work in tandem with other foods, and a few because they are just great-tasting ways to eat better. Our thirty-three-day menu, which begins on page 127, will teach you through repetition how to eat healthfully throughout the day so that by day thirty-four, quality meal planning will be more instinctive than ever.

We will show you the items you need to fill your pantry and fridge, making each shopping list as specific as possible for the foods you'll encounter on the PrayFit Diet each week. This tour through your local supermarket features a lap along the store's outer edges, where you will find the healthiest selections available, such as produce, meats, and cheeses. From there, you'll make a few stops in the heart of the market for products rich in whole grains and heart-healthy oils.

Is eating this way expensive? It doesn't have to be. Another great part of the PrayFit Diet is that it is designed to be workable on any budget. Some will tell you that healthy eating comes at a price, and in the case of some fad diets that may be true. But there are no fancy powders or exotic ingredients to be had here—just whole, healthy food that's available at most supermarkets. You'll still be able to balance your checkbook, even as you are balancing your macronutrients. Dry oats, canned tuna, pasta, and vegetables are all items that are easily found year-round. Eating healthy does not have to break the bank. Financial stewardship counts, too.

All that said, before you hit the market, it's time to do a cleaning (or "leaning") of your pantry, to toss the types of unhealthy foods that aren't a part of the PrayFit Program. Out of sight, out of mind! My advice: take these items out of your house rather than just hiding them away at the back of your fridge or pantry. If you get them out of your home entirely, that's one fewer craving you have to fight.

Speaking of fight, did you know that of all the armor of God that Paul talks about in the Bible, not one item is mentioned to protect us from behind? From the breastplate of righteousness to the shield of faith, God teaches us that we're in for a frontal attack. We'll never be surprised or blindsided. In other words, He's got our backs.

When it comes to our crusade for greater health, most of our fights are frontal, too. The battle comes at us from straight ahead. Whether it be with choices on the lunch menu or setting the alarm early for a morning workout, the blows are before us and in plain sight. Today, decide that your health is worth protecting, starting with your pantry. If you can see it, pick a fight and get rid of it. In doing so, you're that much closer to being armed and ready. And hopefully by the end of your initial thirty-three days on the PrayFit Diet, you'll be feeling so good that you'll want these foods a little less, and the fight won't be so difficult.

Sugary Drinks

You're at an incredibly high risk of weight gain and other health problems if you drink your calories. Many sweetened juices, sodas, and even sweet teas are weighted down in sugars that trigger rapid and considerable releases of insulin, a hormone that tells your body to store fat. Also, these drinks aren't doing your smile any favors, since they tend to promote tooth decay. People who drink a lot of calories—even if they are keeping their food choices reasonable—tend to consume more overall calories than those who drink water instead. Ditch them.

Sugary Cereals

Everything that I've said about sugary drinks holds for sugary cereals as well. Many of us were raised in the era of cartoon-character breakfast cereals that were as brightly colored as they were unhealthy. These sugar-laden puffed wheat cereals pass themselves off as "kid friendly" when in reality they are anything but. Many of them are over 50 percent sugar by weight and are a large contributor to the grim prediction that the current generation of children will be the first to have a shorter life span than their parents. Don't buy them for your kids; don't eat them yourself.

Chips and Popcorn

Are you a late-night snacker? Do you like to have a cauldron of chips next to you for football on Sundays? We all intend to just have a few, but everyone knows how easy it is to lose track of how much you are eating of these salty snacks. And the recommended serving size for most of these unhealthy, processed foods is usually just a few ounces. By the time you hit the bottom of the bowl, you've likely exceeded a day's worth of calories—and not the good kind, either. Toss them.

Prepackaged Muffins

Woe be unto the man who checks the nutrition label on his muffins for the first time. This can be a heavy, saddening revelation for most who have assumed that these quick-breakfast items are relatively harmless. They're not. Just one medium-sized muffin contains over 50 grams of carbohydrates, most of that from simple sugars, and a full 22 grams of greasy, heart-hugging fat. Simple sugars, as we learned, do your body composition no favors, and at 50 grams of them here, one muffin already has taken up a third of your day's carbs. No amount of blueberries is going to make up for that. Store-bought muffins are just cookies by a different name. Don't buy them.

Most Soups

Unless you've made the conscious decision to start shopping healthier already, chances are your soup choices are not the best. While most people consider a good bowl of chicken soup—full of carrots, celery, and the like—to be perfectly healthy, most canned versions are grossly amped on sodium. According to the Mayo Clinic, we should have less than 2,300 mg of sodium a day—or 1,500 mg if you're age fifty-one or older, if you're black, or if you have high blood pressure, diabetes, or chronic kidney disease. A single can of store-bought soup can tax you 700 mg or more in a single serving.

The White Stuff

Bread, tortillas, English muffins, bagels, and buns; the white stuff, the wrong stuff. These products are created using refined flour and fast-digested sugars that do little more than spike your blood sugar. Remember the contrast between slowly digested carbs and quickly digested carbs we discussed in Chapter 3? If it's a white bready food like this, it's almost certainly a fast carb—and we don't want or need those on PrayFit. It's time to wean yourself off them. The good news is that most of these ubiquitous products are available in whole-grain and whole-wheat versions, and those are fair game (in the right serving sizes) for this new way of eating.

Sweets

If it's not in your pantry or fridge, you're that much less likely to eat it, which is why you should get rid of all of your goodie caches. Cookies, cupcakes, donuts, and even most crackers—all of these things are filled with sugar, trans fats, and who knows what else. Most of these foods are full of those dreaded fast-digested carbs—and they have the added detriment of having sugar, too. A better strategy is to get them out of the house and to leave them out of the cart when you shop. We're going to retrain your palate to enjoy less sweetness and more savory tastes on PrayFit.

Meal Replacement Bars

They're at the gas station. They're in your cereal aisle. They're making celebrities thin on television. You can't seem to escape being exposed to meal replacement bars promising rapid weight loss—but you can escape eating them. What? You thought these bars were supposed to be healthy? Think again. There are some healthier options out there for those on-the-go moments when you don't have access to whole foods. (Although really, a piece of fruit is just as easy to stow as a bar in most situations.) But a meal replacement bar should never take the place of whole food.

Unfortunately, a great many of these products are too high in sodium, sugar, fat, and calories to make them good choices for anyone trying to get in better shape.

Mayonnaise

Even if it's low-fat, mayonnaise has very little nutritive value. On PrayFit, you will learn to love other condiments instead. Pass on the mayo.

Deli Meats

Processed meats such as bologna and hot dogs have been linked to a higher risk of heart disease, diabetes, and cancer. They are also calorie bombs oozing with sodium and fat that can set you back a day or more in your weight-loss efforts. I'm going to show you some tastier—and yes, easier—protein alternatives that are leaner, lower in sodium, and altogether more satisfying. Deny the deli meat. (There are exceptions, such as freshly sliced deli turkey and roast beef.)

YOUR JOURNEY STARTS NOW

Over the next thirty-three days, you'll put all this together. You will be using the biblically advocated principle of dietary balance—one that shuns both gluttony and deprivation—in order to achieve the healthiest version of yourself possible. You'll take advantage of the way the various macronutrients (protein, fat, and carbs) work in concert to improve vital health markers while also helping you to lose weight more consistently than ever. You'll capitalize on research that has proven the value of eating equal portions of protein, fat, and carbohydrate, turning lab-tested results into long-term lifestyle choices. And you'll learn exactly what you should be throwing in your shopping cart in order to put the best things possible onto your plate. By day 34, you may very well be *many* pounds lighter, and you will certainly be living more abundantly, just as God intended.

7

WEEK 1

FAITH WORKS

Faith works. But that's the only way it works. As you begin the first week of the PrayFit Diet, I can't help but think of the apostle Paul. He probably understood as well as anyone how critical putting the body under submission was for his life's calling. The last thing Paul would ever let hinder his mission was the body God designed for him to use to accomplish it, and neither should you. If Paul was there with you, reading this over your shoulder, I'd like to humbly think that he would be nodding in agreement. Because not only is faith the most powerful tool God ever gave us to conquer life's obstacles or to fight for our dreams, but it's also the most important reason to conquer or pursue them in the first place. And that includes your health. That includes your food. Yes indeed, Paul knew the power of faith, so he went looking for ways to demonstrate it. You and I need to do the same. And this first week is an excellent opportunity to put your faith to work.

And for your first step of faith, you're going to go shopping. Just as we are trying to redefine your relationship with food in the kitchen, so you should count on redefining your relationship with the market. What you put in your cart ultimately ends up in your belly, so by exercising a bit more discretion—and with our help—you'll be able to confidently stroll the aisles of your local grocery, knowing that your dollar is going toward the body you are building on the PrayFit Diet.

Your mind may be plagued with doubts about your ability to follow through with this diet or to make the changes that are being asked of you, and that's understandable. But that is precisely why this first shopping trip is so important. By touching, feeling, and smelling the body-altering bounty that you are about to enjoy, you are sure to become excited and encouraged at what is to come. You may not buy grapefruits regularly, for example. But when you start looking for delicious ones on this trip and you realize that grapefruit—on its own, without changing anything else—has the potential to start slimming your waistline, that's a bit of a thrill. But guess what? Each item outlined here is going to benefit you, your health, and your weight in one way or another. Taken together, the possibilities are endless. Ladies and gentlemen, start your carts!

WEEK 1 SHOPPING LIST

Produce

Avocados: 2

Oranges: 2

Grapefruit: 3 (The journal *Diabetes* reports that naringenin, a flavonoid found in grapefruit, may possess fat-burning properties. Lab tests showed that naringenin effectively "reprogrammed" the livers of lab mice so that they burned off excess fat instead of storing it.)

Apples: 1

Pomegranates: 2 (Fun, colorful, and good for you. This antioxidant-rich fruit has been shown to lower blood pressure, support immune function, and defend against certain cancers. Remember, only the seeds and juice are edible. Half a cup of seeds also delivers 3 grams of healthy fiber.)

Bananas: 2

Lemons: 3

Berries: 1 pint

Baby spinach: 2 pounds (A potent source of vitamins A, K, D, and E. Spinach also contains carotenoids that aid in eye health and other compounds that function as anticancer agents.)

Cucumbers: 2

Mixed greens: 1 large package (12 cups total)

Broccoli: 2 large bunches (A powerful cancer-fighting food, and it's good for your heart and eyes. Now you can eat it to get healthy—not just because Mom says you have to.)

Zucchini: 1

Tomatoes: 2 large

Baby carrots: 1 bag

Sweet potatoes: 1 (A much more slowly digested choice for your dinner plate, sweet potatoes are high in fiber, vitamin B_6, and potassium.)

Green beans: ½ pound (2 cups)

Cauliflower: 1 large head (One of the primary phytochemicals in cruciferous veggies such as broccoli and cauliflower has been shown to selectively target and kill cancer cells while leaving healthy cells unaffected.)

Dairy and Eggs

Nonfat Greek yogurt: 6 ounces (This versatile food, higher
in protein than traditional yogurt, can be used as a snack,
dessert, or dip.)

Parmesan cheese: 2 tablespoons

Eggs: 1 dozen

Low-fat cheddar cheese: ¼ pound

Cottage cheese: 16 ounces (High in slowly digested casein
protein to keep you feeling full longer, it's also low in carbs
and packed with calcium. What's not to like? Use it as a snack
or as a dip with your veggies.)

Crumbled feta cheese: 1 small container

Part-skim string cheese: 1 small package

Bakery

Ezekiel or whole-wheat tortillas (Lower in calories and higher
in fiber than their white-flour counterpart, this is one of
the easiest, flavor-neutral diet swaps you can make to start
getting lean.)

Ezekiel bread

Ezekiel or whole-wheat English muffins

Meat, Deli, Seafood

Boneless, skinless chicken breast: 2¼ pounds

Chicken thighs: ½ pound

Ground turkey breast: ¾ pound

Flank steak: ⅓ pound

Sliced deli turkey: ¼ pound (Opt for freshly sliced deli turkey
breast over prepackaged sources, and ask the deli attendant
about lower-sodium varieties.)

Salmon: ⅓ pound

Grocery, Pantry

Rolled oats (Each 100-gram serving has 10 grams of dietary
fiber, 16 grams of protein, and a hearty dose of iron and
antioxidants.)

Honey

Almonds

Cinnamon (A great topper for oatmeal, this spice has been
shown to stabilize blood sugar and decrease inflammation
and improve metabolism.)

Walnuts

Shredded coconut (unsweetened)

Extra-virgin olive oil

Balsamic vinegar

Canned tuna

Kalamata olives (This tasty source of healthy fat adds a dash of
Mediterranean flavor to your pantry.)

Bow-tie pasta

Prepared pesto (A flavorful indulgence that can be used to top
light chicken pastas, pesto's main ingredient is olive oil.)

Brown rice

Black beans (One of the best sources of protein and fiber on the
list! A single cup contains 15 grams of each.)

Salsa

Natural peanut butter (Choosing natural over other types helps to
ensure that you avoid any unwanted sugars or unhealthy fats.)

Almond butter

Cumin (This spice provides a flavor boost to many foods, while
also aiding in digestion and stabilizing blood sugar levels.)

Dijon mustard

Frozen

Shelled edamame: 1 bag (Just a half cup of this wonder bean
contains 11 grams of figure-slimming protein.)

WEEK 1 MEAL PLAN

Days 1–7	Day 1	Day 2	Day 3
Breakfast	Honey-Nut Oatmeal Calories: 256 Total Fat: 9 g Saturated Fat: 1 g Carbohydrate: 41 g Protein: 7 g Sodium: 2 mg Cholesterol: 0 mg Fiber: 5 g	4 egg whites, scrambled 1 slice low-fat cheddar cheese 2 slices Ezekiel toast ½ grapefruit Calories: 331 Total Fat: 4 g Saturated Fat: 1 g Carbohydrate: 45 g Protein: 32 g Sodium: 543 mg Cholesterol: 6 mg Fiber: 8 g	1 whole-wheat English muffin 1 tablespoon natural peanut butter 1 cup berries Calories: 318 Total Fat: 10 g Saturated Fat: 2 g Carbohydrate: 51 g Protein: 11 g Sodium: 251 mg Cholesterol: 0 mg Fiber: 7 g
Lunch	5 oz grilled chicken breast ¾ cup cooked brown rice ¾ cup black beans ¼ cup salsa Calories: 620 Total Fat: 8 g Saturated Fat: 2 g Carbohydrate: 79 g Protein: 60 g Sodium: 1,015 mg Cholesterol: 120 mg Fiber: 16 g	Spinach Salad with Walnuts and Pomegranate 3 oz grilled chicken breast 1 banana Calories: 644 Total Fat: 34 g Saturated Fat: 6 g Carbohydrate: 46 g Protein: 46 g Sodium: 653 mg Cholesterol: 108 mg Fiber: 9 g	2 oz deli turkey 2 hard-boiled egg whites 1 cup chopped tomato ¼ chopped avocado 3 cups mixed greens 1 tablespoon olive oil + balsamic vinegar Calories: 321 Total Fat: 12 g Saturated Fat: 2 g Carbohydrate: 19 g Protein: 33 g Sodium: 1,635 mg Cholesterol: 249 mg Fiber: 3 g

Day 4	Day 5	Day 6	Day 7
Breakfast Salad	4 egg whites, scrambled	1 Ezekiel tortilla	Honey-Nut Oatmeal
Calories: 501	1 slice low-fat cheddar cheese	1 tablespoon almond butter	1 orange
Total Fat: 29 g	2 slices Ezekiel toast	1 banana, sliced	
Saturated Fat: 10 g	½ grapefruit		Calories: 434
Carbohydrate: 63 g		Calories: 363	Total Fat: 14 g
Protein: 8 g	Calories: 331	Total Fat: 10 g	Saturated Fat: 3 g
Sodium: 9 mg	Total Fat: 4 g	Saturated Fat: 1 g	Carbohydrate: 66 g
Cholesterol: 0 mg	Saturated Fat: 1 g	Carbohydrate: 60 g	Protein: 16 g
Fiber: 14 g	Carbohydrate: 45 g	Protein: 15 g	Sodium: 68 mg
	Protein: 32 g	Sodium: 151 mg	Cholesterol: 187 mg
	Sodium: 543 mg	Cholesterol: 0 mg	Fiber: 13 g
	Cholesterol: 6 mg	Fiber: 11 g	
	Fiber: 8 g		
5 oz grilled chicken breast	Tuna and Olive Wrap	Spinach Salad with Walnuts and Pomegranate	Turkey Quesadilla (made with 2 Ezekiel tortillas, 2 oz deli turkey, 1 slice low-fat cheddar cheese, Dijon mustard)
1 baked sweet potato topped with ½ cup cooked spinach and 1 tablespoon Greek yogurt	½ cup edamame	4 oz grilled chicken breast	
	Calories: 420		
	Total Fat: 17 g	Calories: 691	
	Saturated Fat: 1 g	Total Fat: 37 g	Calories: 361
Calories: 469	Carbohydrate: 37 g	Saturated Fat: 8 g	Total Fat: 10 g
Total Fat: 5 g	Protein: 36 g	Carbohydrate: 20 g	Saturated Fat: 1 g
Saturated Fat: 1 g	Sodium: 1,099 mg	Protein: 70 g	Carbohydrate: 51 g
Carbohydrate: 54 g	Cholesterol: 38 mg	Sodium: 881 mg	Protein: 19 g
Protein: 50 g	Fiber: 9 g	Cholesterol: 172 mg	Sodium: 576 mg
Sodium: 267 mg		Fiber: 6 g	Cholesterol: 6 mg
Cholesterol: 121 mg			Fiber: 10 g
Fiber: 8 g			

Days 1–7	Day 1	Day 2	Day 3

Snack	1 cup low-fat cottage cheese
	10 baby carrots
	
	Calories: 198
	Total Fat: 2 g
	Saturated Fat : 1 g
	Carbohydrate:
	    14 g
	Protein: 29 g
	Sodium: 996 mg
	Cholesterol: 9 mg
	Fiber: 3 g
		3 tablespoons almonds
		
		Calories: 154
		Total Fat: 13 g
		Saturated Fat: 1 g
		Carbohydrate: 6 g
		Protein: 6 g
		Sodium: 0 mg
		Cholesterol: 0 mg
		Fiber: 3 g
			¾ cup steamed edamame
			
			Calories: 282
			Total Fat: 13 g
			Saturated Fat: 2 g
			Carbohydrate:
			    21 g
			Protein: 25 g
			Sodium: 29 mg
			Cholesterol: 0 mg
			Fiber: 8 g

Dinner	4 oz turkey burger
	3 cups cooked broccoli
	2 tablespoons olive oil and lemon juice
	
	Calories: 594
	Total Fat: 48 g
	Saturated Fat: 9 g
	Carbohydrate:
	    12 g
	Protein: 34 g
	Sodium: 156 mg
	Cholesterol:
	    120 mg
	Fiber: 5 g
		4 oz flank steak
		1 baked sweet potato
		2 cups steamed spinach
		2 tablespoons crumbled feta cheese
		lemon juice
		
		Calories: 481
		Total Fat: 15 g
		Saturated Fat: 7 g
		Carbohydrate:
		    46 g
		Protein: 46 g
		Sodium: 439 mg
		Cholesterol:
		    106 mg
		Fiber: 17 g
			Chicken and Bow Ties
			
			Calories: 691
			Total Fat: 32 g
			Saturated Fat: 7 g
			Carbohydrate:
			    54 g
			Protein: 49 g
			Sodium: 994 mg
			Cholesterol:
			    79 mg
			Fiber: 10 g

Day 4	Day 5	Day 6	Day 7
1 cup low-fat cottage cheese 10 baby carrots Calories: 198 Total Fat: 2 g Saturated Fat: 1 g Carbohydrate: 14 g Protein: 29 g Sodium: 996 mg Cholesterol: 9 mg Fiber: 3 g	1 piece part-skim mozzarella string cheese 1 banana Calories: 185 Total Fat: 6 g Saturated Fat: 4 g Carbohydrate: 27 g Protein: 9 g Sodium: 241 mg Cholesterol: 15 mg Fiber: 3 g	1 grapefruit 1 piece part-skim string cheese Calories: 192 Total Fat: 6 g Saturated Fat: 3 g Carbohydrate: 28 g Protein: 9 g Sodium: 185 mg Cholesterol: 15 mg Fiber: 4 g	1 cup steamed edamame Calories: 180 Total Fat: 8 g Saturated Fat: 2 g Carbohydrate: 14 g Protein: 15 g Sodium: 15 mg Cholesterol: 0 mg Fiber: 5 g
4 oz grilled or roasted salmon 2 cups steamed green beans 1 tablespoon olive oil Calories: 346 Total Fat: 19 g Saturated Fat: 3 g Carbohydrate: 15 g Protein: 31 g Sodium: 79 mg Cholesterol: 62 mg Fiber: 6 g	4 oz turkey burger 3 cups mixed greens ¼ cup chopped avocado 1 tablespoon olive oil + lemon juice Calories: 544 Total Fat: 37 g Saturated Fat: 8 g Carbohydrate: 19 g Protein: 40 g Sodium: 400 mg Cholesterol: 97 mg Fiber: 13 g	4 oz grilled chicken or turkey breast 3 cups cauliflower roasted with 2 teaspoons olive oil and ¼ teaspoon ground cumin Calories: 286 Total Fat: 14 g Saturated Fat: 3 g Carbohydrate: 12 g Protein: 31 g Sodium: 496 mg Cholesterol: 48 mg Fiber: 6 g	4 oz grilled or roasted skinless, boneless chicken thighs 1 cup cooked brown rice 2 cups cooked broccoli 1 tablespoon olive oil lemon juice Calories: 396 Total Fat: 26 g Saturated Fat: 5 g Carbohydrate: 7 g Protein: 34 g Sodium: 138 mg Cholesterol: 108 mg Fiber: 0 g

Days 1–7	Day 1	Day 2	Day 3
Totals for the Day	Calories: 1,668	Calories: 1,610	Calories: 1,612
	Total Fat: 67 g	Total Fat: 65 g	Total Fat: 67 g
	Saturated Fat: 13 g	Saturated Fat: 15 g	Saturated Fat: 12 g
	Carbohydrate: 146 g	Carbohydrate: 142 g	Carbohydrate: 145 g
	Protein: 129 g	Protein: 129 g	Protein: 118 g
	Sodium: 2,169 mg	Sodium: 1,634 mg	Sodium: 2,910 mg
	Cholesterol: 250 mg	Cholesterol: 220 mg	Cholesterol: 328 mg
	Fiber: 29 g	Fiber: 36 g	Fiber: 29 g

• • •

For some of you, week 1 represents both the first step and the longest stride in your quest to a fitter, leaner, healthier you. So, congratulations. It's not easy to make the kinds of changes you've been called to make. For those of you who are accustomed to sugary sodas or donuts, this is undeniably an adjustment. But I

Day 4	Day 5	Day 6	Day 7
Calories: 1,514	Calories: 1,480	Calories: 1,531	Calories: 1,611
Total Fat: 56 g	Total Fat: 64 g	Total Fat: 68 g	Total Fat: 67 g
Saturated Fat: 16 g	Saturated Fat: 14 g	Saturated Fat: 14 g	Saturated Fat: 14 g
Carbohydrate: 147 g	Carbohydrate: 128 g	Carbohydrate: 120 g	Carbohydrate: 138 g
Protein: 117 g	Protein: 117 g	Protein: 126 g	Protein: 122 g
Sodium: 1,351 mg	Sodium: 2,283 mg	Sodium: 1,713 mg	Sodium: 858 mg
Cholesterol: 193 mg	Cholesterol: 156 mg	Cholesterol: 235 mg	Cholesterol: 414 mg
Fiber: 31 g	Fiber: 33 g	Fiber: 26 g	Fiber: 28 g

pray you are already feeling as healthy in body as you are strong in spirit. Nobody sees what's motivating you to eat healthier, so if they ask why the change in heart toward food, health, and the zest for life, just tell them it's for Heaven's sake. And for Heaven's sake, tell them faith works. But that's the *only* way it works.

WEEK 1

Congratulations for taking the first step. How are you feeling after this week?

_____

_____

Were the shopping lists helpful? What adjustments if any did you choose to make?

_____

_____

What was your favorite breakfast?

_____

_____

Is making breakfast a habit or something new to you? In just over a week, do you feel a difference in your productivity because of the balanced first meal of the day?

_____

_____

What were your challenges this week? Did you skip any meals? Which ones?

_____

_____

Did you prepare some meals in advance? Which ones?

_____

_____

Did other members of your household enjoy some or all of the meals you prepared?

_____

_____

Did you make any modifications or adjustments to best meet your needs, tastes, or schedule? What were they and why?

_____

_____

How is your energy level? Are you feeling more energized at work, at school, or at play?

_____

_____

Do you notice any physical changes—do your clothes fit better? Have you seen any results on the scale? What other by-products of obedience and diligence are you measuring? Blood pressure? Waist-hip girth?

_____

_____

Do you anticipate any challenges next week (parties, trips, time away from home)? How will you plan ahead to work through those challenges?

_____

_____

What were some moments of success you experienced this week? What about moments of weakness? Did you give in to certain cravings and desires?

_____

_____

How can you bring those moments of success into next week? And how will you overcome the moments of weakness next week?

_____

_____

How has your faith helped you through tough times this first week? Did you experience any doubts and fears? How did your faith see you through? Did you put your faith to work?

_____

_____

Are you spending quality time alone with God? Do you feel connected with the Lord? As you're becoming more fit physically, what do you need to do to grow more spiritually?

_____

_____

Have you shared your spiritual and physical goals with a trusted friend? Is he or she holding you accountable?

_____

_____

For some of you, this first week represented the first step and longest stride. Congratulations. How does it feel to know you're that much closer to your goals?

_____

_____

How does it feel to be eating in a way that allows you to be a better steward of your health?

_____

_____

If you were to achieve all of your physical goals, what will you do for the cause of Christ with your health? Be specific.

_____

_____

COMMITMENT: This week is over, and I'm thankful for each triumph and for what I learned through each pitfall. Looking ahead to next week, I commit to the Lord, myself, and my family that I will_____ in week 2 in order to live a healthier, more active, and abundant life.

PRAYER: *Lord, I love you and thank you for my health. Help me trust you with each day, putting my heart and my life in your hands. Give me the strength I need to meet today's needs, and I thank you for the food that will fuel me to that end. I give you all the glory, honor, and praise. In Jesus' name, I pray, amen.*

8

WEEK 2

NO TURNING BACK

The story of Moses leading the Israelites out of bondage in Egypt is a familiar one to most of us. But one small verse sure packs a punch for you and for me here in week 2. In Numbers 11:20, the Israelites say, "Why did we ever leave Egypt?" Yes, they actually *missed* captivity. Not long after the Israelites met freedom, they actually longed for captivity. That's right. As captives, they had no choices, no responsibility. Even though they were trapped, they were warm, cozy, safe, and full of food. Their prayer for freedom was a dangerous one. Once they were set free, the Israelites faced the need for *obedience* and *responsibility*—nothing a generation in the desert couldn't answer.

What about us? When was the last time you and I prayed dangerously? About finances, a relationship . . . our health, better food? The fact that you're reading and studying this book means you have prayed a similar prayer. You're desperate to be free from the prison of food guilt, of poor choices, of a sedentary lifestyle. And like the Israelites, you're face-to-face with obedience and responsibility. But thankfully, our bodies are merely tools, not finished products. Better food simply means being better equipped. It's tough to visit the poor from the couch, and it's impossible to see the hurting if we're stuck looking in our own mirror.

As you begin week 2, you may be thinking to yourself, "Why did I ever leave Egypt? Why did I start eating healthier? Why did I clean my pantry out?" You may have thoughts like that, and that's all right. After all, like the Israelites, you were warm, cozy, and full.

But press on. If God allows you the opportunity for better health because of what and how you eat in week 2, just remind yourself of what you'll do with it. Let the thought of a slimmer, healthier version stir your heart and jog your memory. We know why the Israelites left Egypt, and we know why you did, too.

WEEK 2 SHOPPING LIST

Produce

Lemons: 2

Red apple: 1

Green apple: 1

Berries: 1 quart

Grapefruit: 2

Kale: 1 bunch

Fresh basil

Fresh rosemary

Fresh ginger (This unsightly herb tastes better than it looks and is used to treat everything from motion sickness to migraines. But it also enhances the inflammation-reduction benefits of the PrayFit Diet.)

Fresh tarragon: 1 bunch (This will be a key ingredient in one of the more savory recipes on the PrayFit Diet but it can be used to add more flavor, vitamins, and minerals to many dishes.)

Green cabbage: 1 head

Large carrots: 1 medium

Baby carrots: 1 bag

Leeks: 2 large (A relative of the onion, leeks are known to aid in circulation and heart health.)

Mushrooms: 1 cup

Tomatoes: 2

Asparagus: 1 bunch

Sweet potato: 1

Broccoli: 1 large bunch

Mixed greens: 1 package (6 cups total)

Green beans: ½ pound (2 cups)

Cucumber: 1

Dairy and Eggs

Nonfat Greek yogurt: 16 ounces

2% plain Greek yogurt: 6 ounces

2% flavored Greek yogurt: 2.5 cups

Provolone cheese: ¼ pound (A perfect sandwich topper, provolone is also relatively high in protein. Shred for pizza toppings or slice for sandwiches.)

Part-skim shredded mozzarella: ¼ cup

Part-skim string cheese: 1 small package

Swiss cheese: 2 ounces

Eggs: 1 dozen (The benefits of eggs don't have to stop when breakfast is over. Hard-boiled eggs make a great snack—easy, quick, high in protein, and self-packaged.)

Crumbled blue cheese: ¼ cup

1% milk or soy milk: 1 gallon

Crumbled feta cheese: ¼ cup (Great on salads, this type of cheese is full of fat-fighting calcium.)

Bakery

Whole-wheat pizza dough: 8 ounces (Pizza doesn't have to be off-limits. Starting with a whole-wheat crust allows you to build a healthier pie.)

Ezekiel bread (A complete source of protein and a healthier alternative to white or wheat bread.)

Ezekiel tortillas

Meat, Deli, Seafood

Boneless pork chops: 1 pound

Boneless, skinless chicken breast: 2½ pounds

Ground turkey breast: ½ pound

Deli turkey: 6 ounces

Flank steak: ⅓ pound (A tasty, less commonly eaten red meat that won't send your calorie intake through the roof.)

Salmon: ⅓ pound

Grocery, Pantry

Green tea (Dumped into your smoothie, green tea adds flavor without adding too many calories. Also, it's rich in antioxidants and a fat-fighting compound called EGCG, epigallocatechin gallate.)

Honey

Whole-grain cereal (Time to ditch the Froot Loops in favor of some fiber-rich whole grains. Look for brands that are low in sugar and high in fiber to ensure you get the waist-slimming benefits.)

Canned chickpeas (Use as a side or puree into hummus. Full of fiber and protein, chickpeas also contain tryptophan, which aids in sleep.)

Sesame tahini

Smoked paprika

Tomato sauce

Celery salt

Honey

Canned artichoke hearts

Chicken broth

Sliced almonds

Whole almonds

Ground flaxseed (This healthy fat can be used in baking or to
    amp up your Greek yogurt and smoothies.)

Almond butter

Honey mustard

Brown rice

Rice wine vinegar

Minestrone soup (This veggie-filled Italian mainstay can aid in
    fat loss and overall health. Choose low-sodium.)

Balsamic vinegar

Frozen

Frozen mango chunks: 1 bag (4 cups total)

Shelled edamame: 1 bag

Until you found this book, you've been doing everything you can to lose weight or gain better health, but to no avail. And if there's one thing I personally ask or even implore you to do, it's to keep striving. If you're like me, you can relate to Peter, who in one moment declares adamantly that he will *never* deny he knows who Jesus is; the next, he does it not once, not twice, but thrice. But still, what motivates me about Peter is that while he wasn't perfect, he was the one who stepped up. He wasn't always *right*, but he was never in *doubt*. First to reach for his sword to defend the Lord (only to be taught a quick lesson in self-control), and first to get out of the boat (only to be the example of how we sink without faith). But there was a common thread to the life of Peter: the more often he was first to fall, the more he learned to stand.

WEEK 2 MEAL PLAN

Days 8–14	Day 1	Day 2	Day 3
Breakfast	Mango Green Tea Smoothie Calories: 305 Total Fat: 1 g Saturated Fat: 0 g Carbohydrate: 67 g Protein: 12 g Sodium: 63 mg Cholesterol: 7 mg Fiber: 5 g	1 cup nonfat Greek yogurt 2 tablespoons sliced almonds 1 tablespoon ground flaxseed 1 cup berries Calories: 392 Total Fat: 16 g Saturated Fat: 1 g Carbohydrate: 38 g Protein: 31 g Sodium: 95 mg Cholesterol: 0 mg Fiber: 9 g	2 slices Ezekiel toast 2 tablespoons almond butter ½ grapefruit Calories: 408 Total Fat: 18 g Saturated Fat: 1 g Carbohydrate: 49 g Protein: 19 g Sodium: 150 mg Cholesterol: 0 mg Fiber: 11 g
Lunch	Vegetable Pizza (make 2, with different toppings, for another lunch on Day 4) Calories: 524 Total Fat: 32 g Saturated Fat: 16 g Carbohydrate: 32 g Protein: 36 g Sodium: 2,379 mg Cholesterol: 75 mg Fiber: 6 g	3 oz deli turkey 1 slice Swiss cheese 3 slices avocado Sliced tomato 2 slices Ezekiel bread Calories: 459 Total Fat: 17 g Saturated Fat: 5 g Carbohydrate: 42 g Protein: 33 g Sodium: 1,748 mg Cholesterol: 87 mg Fiber: 7 g	5 oz grilled chicken breast ½ cup cooked brown rice 2 cups steamed broccoli 2 tablespoons honey mustard Calories: 398 Total Fat: 6 g Saturated Fat: 2 g Carbohydrate: 33 g Protein: 50 g Sodium: 234 mg Cholesterol: 120 mg Fiber: 2 g

Day 4	Day 5	Day 6	Day 7
1 cup nonfat Greek yogurt	Mango Green Tea Smoothie	2 cups whole-grain cereal	2 slices Ezekiel toast
2 tablespoons sliced almonds	Calories: 305	1 cup milk or soy milk	2 tablespoons almond butter
1 tablespoon ground flaxseed	Total Fat: 1 g	½ cup berries	1 grapefruit
1 cup berries	Saturated Fat: 0 g		
	Carbohydrate: 67 g	Calories: 391	Calories: 428
Calories: 326	Protein: 12 g	Total Fat: 5 g	Total Fat: 18 g
Total Fat: 11 g	Sodium: 63 mg	Saturated Fat: 0 g	Saturated Fat: 1 g
Saturated Fat: 1 g	Cholesterol: 7 mg	Carbohydrate: 44 g	Carbohydrate: 34 g
Carbohydrate: 36 g	Fiber: 5 g	Protein: 11 g	Protein: 14 g
Protein: 28 g		Sodium: 132 mg	Sodium: 75 mg
Sodium: 95 mg		Cholesterol: 5 mg	Cholesterol: 0 mg
Cholesterol: 0 mg		Fiber: 2 g	Fiber: 8 g
Fiber: 8 g			
Vegetable Pizza	2 cups low-sodium minestrone or black bean soup	3 oz deli turkey or roast beef	4 oz grilled chicken or turkey breast
Calories: 463	1 piece part-skim string cheese	1 slice Swiss cheese	1 cup chopped tomato
Total Fat: 29 g		3 slices avocado	3 cups mixed greens
Saturated Fat: 16 g		Sliced tomato	¼ cup crumbled feta cheese
Carbohydrate: 17 g	Calories: 540	2 slices Ezekiel bread	1 tablespoon olive oil + balsamic vinegar
Protein: 33 g	Total Fat: 16 g		
Sodium: 1,573 mg	Saturated Fat: 2 g	Calories: 496	
Cholesterol: 75 mg	Carbohydrate: 75 g	Total Fat: 19 g	Calories: 471
Fiber: 4 g	Protein: 37 g	Saturated Fat: 5 g	Total Fat: 27 g
	Sodium: 255 mg	Carbohydrate: 38 g	Saturated Fat: 8 g
	Cholesterol: 10 mg	Protein: 36 g	Carbohydrate: 25 g
	Fiber: 15 g	Sodium: 1,067 mg	Protein: 40 g
		Cholesterol: 56 mg	Sodium: 635 mg
		Fiber: 7 g	Cholesterol: 107 mg
			Fiber: 14 g

Days 8–14	Day 1	Day 2	Day 3

Snack	1 hard-boiled egg
	
	Calories: 78
	Total Fat: 5 g
	Saturated Fat: 2 g
	Carbohydrate: 1 g
	Protein: 6 g
	Sodium: 62 mg
	Cholesterol:
	  187 mg
	Fiber: 0 g
		¼ cup Hummus
		10 baby carrots
		
		Calories: 170
		Total Fat: 9 g
		Saturated Fat: 1 g
		Carbohydrate:
		  21 g
		Protein: 4 g
		Sodium: 312 mg
		Cholesterol: 0 mg
		Fiber: 5 g
			1 hard-boiled egg
			2 tablespoons
			  almonds
			
			Calories: 180
			Total Fat: 14 g
			Saturated Fat: 2 g
			Carbohydrate: 4 g
			Protein: 10 g
			Sodium: 62 mg
			Cholesterol:
			  187 mg
			Fiber: 2 g

Dinner	Chicken
	  Jerusalem
	  (make a
	  double batch
	  for dinner on
	  day 5)
	
	Calories: 543
	Total Fat: 18 g
	Saturated Fat: 3 g
	Carbohydrate:
	  26 g
	Protein: 61 g
	Sodium: 1,817 mg
	Cholesterol:
	  131 mg
	Fiber: 11 g
		5 oz grilled flank
		  steak or beef
		  tenderloin
		2 cups roasted
		  asparagus
		1 oz crumbled
		  blue cheese
		1 baked sweet
		  potato
		
		Calories: 601
		Total Fat: 27 g
		Saturated Fat:
		  13 g
		Carbohydrate:
		  37 g
		Protein: 54 g
		Sodium: 574 mg
		Cholesterol:
		  122 mg
		Fiber: 10 g
			Pork Chops with
			  Apple Slaw
			  (make an extra
			  pork chop for
			  day 4)
			
			Calories: 542
			Total Fat: 19 g
			Saturated Fat: 1 g
			Carbohydrate:
			  43 g
			Protein: 52 g
			Sodium: 4,907 mg
			Cholesterol:
			  156 mg
			Fiber: 8 g

Day 4	Day 5	Day 6	Day 7

¼ cup Hummus
1 Ezekiel tortilla
 	
Calories: 210
Total Fat: 9 g
Saturated Fat: 1 g
Carbohydrate:
  28 g
Protein: 6 g
Sodium: 385 mg
Cholesterol: 0 mg
Fiber: 5 g
	1 medium apple
	2 tablespoons
	  peanut or
	  almond butter
	
	Calories: 280
	Total Fat: 16 g
	Saturated Fat: 1 g
	Carbohydrate: 28 g
	Protein: 4 g
	Sodium: 2 mg
	Cholesterol: 0 mg
	Fiber: 6 g
		2 hard-boiled eggs
		
		Calories: 156
		Total Fat: 10 g
		Saturated Fat: 4 g
		Carbohydrate: 2 g
		Protein: 12 g
		Sodium: 124 mg
		Cholesterol:
		  250 mg
		Fiber: 0 g
			¼ cup Hummus
			10 pieces sliced
			  cucumber
			
			Calories: 143
			Total Fat: 9 g
			Saturated Fat: 1 g
			Carbohydrate:
			  14 g
			Protein: 3 g
			Sodium: 236 mg
			Cholesterol: 0 mg
			Fiber: 3 g

4 oz leftover pork
  chop
3 cups mixed
  greens
½ cup chickpeas
¼ cup edamame
Ginger Dressing:
  1 tablespoon
  olive oil,
  1 tablespoon
  rice wine
  vinegar,
  1 teaspoon
  honey,
  ⅛ teaspoon
  grated fresh
  ginger
 	
Calories: 508
Total Fat: 13 g
Saturated Fat: 3 g
Carbohydrate: 51 g
Protein: 50 g
Sodium: 662 mg
Cholesterol: 95 mg
Fiber: 23 g
	Chicken
	  Jerusalem
	
	Calories: 543
	Total Fat: 18 g
	Saturated Fat: 3 g
	Carbohydrate:
	  26 g
	Protein: 61 g
	Sodium: 1,817 mg
	Cholesterol:
	  131 mg
	Fiber: 11 g
		5 oz grilled turkey
		  burger
		2 cups steamed
		  green beans
		Frozen Greek
		  Yogurt
		
		Calories: 501
		Total Fat: 20 g
		Saturated Fat: 5 g
		Carbohydrate:
		  25 g
		Protein: 42 g
		Sodium: 110 mg
		Cholesterol:
		  120 mg
		Fiber: 6 g
			5 oz roasted
			  salmon
			3 cups kale
			  sautéed in
			  1 tablespoon
			  olive oil and
			  balsamic
			  vinegar)
			1 baked sweet
			  potato
			
			Calories: 502
			Total Fat: 24 g
			Saturated Fat: 1 g
			Carbohydrate:
			  31 g
			Protein: 38 g
			Sodium: 147 mg
			Cholesterol:
			  62 mg
			Fiber: 8 g

Days 8–14	Day 1	Day 2	Day 3
Totals for the Day	Calories: 1,449	Calories: 1,622	Calories: 1,528
	Total Fat: 57 g	Total Fat: 69 g	Total Fat: 58 g
	Saturated Fat: 21 g	Saturated Fat: 21 g	Saturated Fat: 6 g
	Carbohydrate: 126 g	Carbohydrate: 139 g	Carbohydrate: 130 g
	Protein: 115 g	Protein: 121 g	Protein: 131 g
	Sodium: 4,321 mg	Sodium: 2,730 mg	Sodium: 5,353 mg
	Cholesterol: 400 mg	Cholesterol: 209 mg	Cholesterol: 463 mg
	Fiber: 22 g	Fiber: 31 g	Fiber: 23 g

In your pursuit of a stronger faith, as well as better health, you've likely made bold declarations that you'll pray more and eat better, only to do the exact opposite the next moment. But take courage. *Keep* being first. Because you're attacking week 2 of this lifelong plan, you're setting the pace with your family and

Day 4	Day 5	Day 6	Day 7
Calories: 1,506	Calories: 1,668	Calories: 1,544	Calories: 1,544
Total Fat: 62 g	Total Fat: 51 g	Total Fat: 54 g	Total Fat: 85 g
Saturated Fat: 21 g	Saturated Fat: 5 g	Saturated Fat: 16 g	Saturated Fat: 12 g
Carbohydrate: 132 g	Carbohydrate: 186 g	Carbohydrate: 109 g	Carbohydrate: 104 g
Protein: 117 g	Protein: 114 g	Protein: 101 g	Protein: 95 g
Sodium: 2,715 mg	Sodium: 2,137 mg	Sodium: 1,711 mg	Sodium: 1,092 mg
Cholesterol: 171 mg	Cholesterol: 148 mg	Cholesterol: 383 mg	Cholesterol: 169 mg
Fiber: 39 g	Fiber: 37 g	Fiber: 16 g	Fiber: 32 g

friends. Remember, Peter knows what it's like to declare and fail, to step out and sink. Pursuing obedience is a *staggering* undertaking. Fortunately, like Peter the pacesetter, we have a Savior who reaches further than the fall. And that's why—He's why—we pick ourselves up and keep going.

WEEK 2

How are you feeling this second week?

_____

_____

Name some successes, big and small. What do you have to do to ensure you repeat them and improve upon them?

_____

_____

Do you notice any physical changes—do your clothes fit better, have you seen any results on the scale?

_____

_____

Name some of the pitfalls and setbacks you faced. Could they have been avoided? What steps will you take this next week to avoid them?

_____

_____

How did the meal prep go? What were your challenges this week? Did you skip any meals? Which ones?

_____

_____

Did you prepare some meals in advance? Which ones?

_____

_____

Did other members of your household enjoy some or all of the meals you prepared?

_____

_____

What was your favorite lunch?

_____

_____

Now that you're becoming familiar with the PrayFit plate, what modifications or variations or combinations are you creating that work well with your taste or schedule?

_____

_____

How has your improved eating pattern affected your focus throughout the day? Are you a student? Housewife? Stay-at-home dad? Teacher? Construction worker? No matter your job title, how has the balanced meal plan helped you at your God-given daily tasks?

_____

_____

We know that the Israelites complained after they were set free from bondage. They even longed to be back in captivity where there was no need for discipline and trust. Can you relate to them this week? Are you missing your old habits? How is your faith helping remind you why you're eating better?

_____

_____

Does the thought of a slimmer, healthier, and more active version of "_you_" help you put one foot in front of the other? Knowing God provided for Moses and the Israelites, do you trust that God is providing for you?

_____

_____

If you felt like giving up, how have you depended on the Lord for strength? And how has it helped your family and friends? Is someone you know and love depending on you to succeed in becoming healthier? Who is it?

_____

_____

COMMITMENT: I am grateful and thankful for the first step I've taken to give God control of my health. Although the adjustment was a shock, I won't look back. I will keep putting one foot in front of the other. This week, I commit to the Lord, myself, and my family that I will _____ in week 3 in order to live a healthier, more active, and abundant life.

PRAYER: *Lord, I praise you and thank you for who you are and for seeing beyond my faults and meeting my real needs. I love you because you first loved me. I thank you for another glorious week to serve you with my health; health that begins at the table that only you can fill. In Jesus' name, amen.*

9

WEEK 3

HIS HANDIWORK

The song of creation. Can you hear it? You and I are God's special guests in a masterpiece performed in His honor that He conducts. Not only that, He's given us first chair. In orchestra-speak, first chair is reserved for the one who is both most capable and responsible, regardless of the instrument played. You and I are active participants in a grand arrangement entitled "Creation." When the Pharisees demanded that Jesus quiet the praise of His disciples, He assured them that if the disciples hushed, they would hear "rock" music. And it's with that underlying theme that you begin week 3. We have a timeless reminder of those Hands that made us and which we live in. That's why you're about to reach for the foods in week 3 of the PrayFit Diet. Your hands won't rest until you've completed your journey, especially knowing that God didn't rest His until He completed you and me and said we were good.

This week you should be feeling the rush of energy through your entire body, all the way down to your very core. The confidence you've gained by renewing your mind toward food and pushing through the critical first two weeks is starting to show, even physically. The scale is likely showcasing your efforts, but the most stirring testament is your overall approach to food, the knowledge of serving sizes, and the satiety provided by properly timed portions.

Friends, as you begin building your PrayFit Plate this week, remember that the God of wonder, who has a beyond-conceivable love and unbelievable future for us, is worthy to be praised with everything we have: our minds, our money, our time, and, yes, our bodies. The song of creation—are you playing it? It's your life. Your cue! You *can't* be silent. He gave you the music. You *are* the music. Just read the notes and watch the Master. You're in the first chair. Be amazed . . . and play.

WEEK 3 SHOPPING LIST

Produce

Oranges: 4

Bananas: 2

Grapefruit: 3

Pineapple: 1 small

Berries: 1 pint (Antioxidant-rich picks such as blueberries and raspberries work best. One animal study showed that rats had significantly less belly fat, lower blood fats, lower cholesterol, and improved blood sugar and insulin levels when consuming more blueberries.)

Apples: 2

Lemons: 3

Beets: 2 (An underappreciated superfood that combats colon cancer, boosts heart health, and packs a strong fiber punch.)

Baby spinach: 1 pound

Carrots: 2 large

English cucumber: 1

Tomatoes: 1¼ pounds

Bell pepper: 1

Yellow onions: 1

Baby carrots: 1 bag

Garlic: 1 head (There's not much garlic doesn't do. In addition to aiding in heart health and fighting off cancer, it is a flavorful addition to many dishes.)

Cauliflower: 1 large head

Spaghetti squash: 1 large

Mixed greens: 1 package (6 cups total)

Broccoli: 2 bunches

Sweet potato: 1

Dairy and Eggs

Goat cheese: 2 ounces

Nonfat Greek yogurt: 2.5 cups

Eggs: 1 dozen

Low-fat cheddar cheese: ¼ pound

Low-fat cottage cheese: 16 ounces

Skim milk: ½ gallon

Crumbled feta: ¼ cup

Part-skim string cheese: 1 small package

Shredded cheddar cheese: 2 ounces

Bakery

Whole-wheat English muffins (High in fiber and a welcome change from your usual morning toast. Slather in natural peanut butter or almond butter for a protein-rich snack.)

Ezekiel tortillas

Ezekiel bread

Meat, Deli, Seafood

Ground turkey breast: 1½ pounds

Deli roast beef: ½ pound

Deli turkey: ¼ pound

Boneless, skinless chicken breast: 1¼ pounds

Salmon: ¾ pound

Boneless, skinless chicken thighs: ½ pound

Flank steak: ⅓ pound

Grocery, Pantry

Rolled oats

Sliced almonds

Sweetened shredded coconut

Maple syrup (Go for good ol' real maple syrup instead of the
sugar-free brands, which may contain harmful synthetics. Plus,
real maple syrup is loaded with immune-boosting zinc and
manganese, which ensures you'll be able to continue training
toward your goals. It's used as part of a granola recipe in week
3, so you won't have to worry about it spiking your insulin.)

Dried apricots

Tomato juice

Red wine vinegar

Semisweet chocolate chips

Oregano

Fennel seed

Crushed tomatoes

Natural peanut butter

Almonds

Whole-grain crackers (Sometimes you just need a crunch.
Whole-grain crackers provide a snacky interlude while still
providing you a dose of much-needed whole grain.)

Cumin

Brown rice

Black beans

Salsa

Balsamic vinegar

Almond butter

Fruit jam

Marinara sauce

Frozen

Shelled edamame: 1 bag

WEEK 3 MEAL PLAN

Days 15–21	Day 1	Day 2	Day 3
Breakfast	½ cup Coconut-Apricot Granola 1 cup nonfat Greek yogurt 1 orange Calories: 440 Total Fat: 9 g Saturated Fat: 3 g Carbohydrate: 67 g Protein: 27 g Sodium: 140 mg Cholesterol: 0 mg Fiber: 11 g	2 eggs 1 whole-wheat English muffin 1 tablespoon natural peanut butter 1 banana Calories: 415 Total Fat: 11 g Saturated Fat: 2 g Carbohydrate: 64 g Protein: 18 g Sodium: 336 mg Cholesterol: 0 mg Fiber: 8 g	½ cup Coconut-Apricot Granola 1½ cups nonfat Greek yogurt Calories: 401 Total Fat: 9 g Saturated Fat: 3 g Carbohydrate: 47 g Protein: 39 g Sodium: 165 mg Cholesterol: 23 mg Fiber: 4 g
Lunch	1 Ezekiel tortilla 3 oz deli roast beef 1 slice low-fat cheddar cheese Sliced tomato Dijon mustard 1 grapefruit Calories: 401 Total Fat: 8 g Saturated Fat: 2 g Carbohydrate: 50 g Protein: 34 g Sodium: 888 mg Cholesterol: 66 mg Fiber: 8 g	Roasted Beet Salad 3 oz grilled chicken Calories: 489 Total Fat: 26 g Saturated Fat: 9 g Carbohydrate: 26 g Protein: 39 g Sodium: 441 mg Cholesterol: 95 mg Fiber: 8 g	Leftover Gazpacho 2 slices Ezekiel bread 2 oz low-fat cheddar cheese Calories: 467 Total Fat: 20 g Saturated Fat: 10 g Carbohydrate: 46 g Protein: 26 g Sodium: 1,092 mg Cholesterol: 40 mg Fiber: 11 g

Day 4	Day 5	Day 6	Day 7
1 cup cooked oatmeal (made with milk or soy milk) 1 cup berries	1 Ezekiel tortilla 1 tablespoon almond butter ½ banana, sliced	¾ cup Coconut-Apricot Granola 1 cup skim milk ½ grapefruit	1 cup cooked oatmeal (made with milk or soy milk) 2 eggs (any style)
Calories: 323 Total Fat: 7 g Saturated Fat: 1 g Carbohydrate: 53 g Protein: 13 g Sodium: 125 mg Cholesterol: 0 mg Fiber: 7 g	Calories: 300 Total Fat: 12 g Saturated Fat: 1 g Carbohydrate: 40 g Protein: 11 g Sodium: 141 mg Cholesterol: 0 mg Fiber: 8 g	Calories: 466 Total Fat: 14 g Saturated Fat: 4 g Carbohydrate: 75 g Protein: 17 g Sodium: 180 mg Cholesterol: 5 mg Fiber: 8 g	Calories: 391 Total Fat: 14 g Saturated Fat: 4 g Carbohydrate: 40 g Protein: 26 g Sodium: 252 mg Cholesterol: 378 mg Fiber: 4 g
5 oz grilled chicken breast ½ cup cooked brown rice ½ cup black beans ¼ cup salsa	Roasted Beet Salad 4 oz grilled chicken or salmon	1 Ezekiel tortilla 3 oz deli roast beef 1 slice low-fat cheddar cheese Sliced tomato Dijon mustard 1 grapefruit	1 slice Ezekiel bread 3 tablespoons natural peanut butter 1 tablespoon jam
Calories: 510 Total Fat: 7 g Saturated Fat: 2 g Carbohydrate: 47 g Protein: 62 g Sodium: 797 mg Cholesterol: 145 mg Fiber: 11 g	Calories: 536 Total Fat: 27 g Saturated Fat: 9 g Carbohydrate: 26 g Protein: 48 g Sodium: 462 mg Cholesterol: 119 mg Fiber: 8 g	Calories: 401 Total Fat: 8 g Saturated Fat: 2 g Carbohydrate: 50 g Protein: 34 g Sodium: 888 mg Cholesterol: 66 mg Fiber: 8 g	Calories: 415 Total Fat: 25 g Saturated Fat: 4 g Carbohydrate: 39 g Protein: 16 g Sodium: 210 mg Cholesterol: 0 mg Fiber: 6 g

Days 15–21	Day 1	Day 2	Day 3

Snack	¼ cup almonds
	1 hard-boiled egg
	
	Calories: 283
	Total Fat: 23 g
	Saturated Fat: 3 g
	Carbohydrate: 8 g
	Protein: 14 g
	Sodium: 62 mg
	Cholesterol:
	  187 mg
	Fiber: 4 g
		1 cup low-fat
		  cottage cheese
		½ cup chopped
		  pineapple
		10 baby carrots
		
		Calories: 239
		Total Fat: 3 g
		Saturated Fat: 1 g
		Carbohydrate:
		  25 g
		Protein: 29 g
		Sodium: 996 mg
		Cholesterol: 9 mg
		Fiber: 4 g
			1 cup steamed
			  edamame
			1 apple
			
			Calories: 296
			Total Fat: 8 g
			Saturated Fat: 2 g
			Carbohydrate:
			  44 g
			Protein: 16 g
			Sodium: 17 mg
			Cholesterol: 0 mg
			Fiber: 10 g

Dinner	5 oz grilled or
	  roasted tuna or
	  salmon
	3 cups cauliflower
	  roasted with
	  1 tablespoon
	  olive oil and
	  ¼ teaspoon
	  cumin
	
	Calories: 420
	Total Fat: 22 g
	Saturated Fat: 4 g
	Carbohydrate: 12 g
	Protein: 46 g
	Sodium: 145 mg
	Cholesterol:
	  94 mg
	Fiber: 6 g
		Gazpacho
		5 whole-grain
		  crackers
		5 oz grilled
		  or roasted
		  skinless,
		  boneless
		  chicken thighs
		
		Calories: 542
		Total Fat: 27 g
		Saturated Fat: 7 g
		Carbohydrate:
		  25 g
		Protein: 49 g
		Sodium: 832 mg
		Cholesterol: 162
		  mg
		Fiber: 5 g
			5 oz cooked
			  turkey burger
			3 cups mixed
			  greens
			¼ cup crumbled
			  feta
			1 tablespoon olive
			  oil + lemon
			  juice
			
			Calories: 516
			Total Fat: 24 g
			Saturated Fat:
			  8 g
			Carbohydrate:
			  20 g
			Protein: 57 g
			Sodium: 596 mg
			Cholesterol:
			  138 mg
			Fiber: 13 g

Day 4	Day 5	Day 6	Day 7

½ cup low-fat cottage cheese
¼ cup almonds
 	
Calories: 287
Total Fat: 19 g
Saturated Fat: 2 g
Carbohydrate:
  11 g
Protein: 22 g
Sodium: 459 mg
Cholesterol: 5 mg
Fiber: 4 g
	1 piece part-skim string cheese
	1 apple
	
	Calories: 175
	Total Fat: 6 g
	Saturated Fat: 4 g
	Carbohydrate:
	  25 g
	Protein: 8 g
	Sodium: 242 mg
	Cholesterol:
	  15 mg
	Fiber: 4 g
		¼ cup almonds
		
		Calories: 206
		Total Fat: 18 g
		Saturated Fat: 1 g
		Carbohydrate: 8 g
		Protein: 8 g
		Sodium: 0 mg
		Cholesterol: 0 mg
		Fiber: 4 g
			1 cup steamed edamame
			3 slices deli turkey
			
			Calories: 275
			Total Fat: 10 g
			Saturated Fat: 2 g
			Carbohydrate:
			  20 g
			Protein: 26 g
			Sodium: 1,036 mg
			Cholesterol:
			  47 mg
			Fiber: 5 g

Turkey Meat Sauce
2 cups cooked spaghetti squash
2 cups baby spinach
1 tablespoon olive oil + balsamic vinegar
 	
Calories: 507
Total Fat: 22 g
Saturated Fat: 3 g
Carbohydrate:
  43 g
Protein: 37 g
Sodium: 603 mg
Cholesterol:
  71 mg
Fiber: 12 g
	5 oz flank steak
	1 baked sweet potato
	3 cups mixed greens
	1 tablespoon balsamic vinaigrette
	
	Calories: 591
	Total Fat: 19 g
	Saturated Fat: 6 g
	Carbohydrate:
	  49 g
	Protein: 59 g
	Sodium: 443 mg
	Cholesterol:
	  133 mg
	Fiber: 17 g
		6 oz grilled or roasted chicken breast
		2 cups cooked broccoli
		Lemon juice
		Chocolate-Dipped Oranges
		
		Calories: 531
		Total Fat: 19 g
		Saturated Fat: 7 g
		Carbohydrate:
		  33 g
		Protein: 59 g
		Sodium: 164 mg
		Cholesterol:
		  145 mg
		Fiber: 3 g
			Turkey Meat Sauce Pizza
			1 Ezekiel tortilla topped with
			¼ cup marinara sauce
			¼ cup shredded cheese (bake until cheese is melted)
			
			Calories: 539
			Total Fat: 18 g
			Saturated Fat: 4 g
			Carbohydrate:
			  49 g
			Protein: 46 g
			Sodium: 1,071 mg
			Cholesterol:
			  89 mg
			Fiber: 11 g

Days 15–21	Day 1	Day 2	Day 3
Totals for the Day	Calories: 1,543	Calories: 1,685	Calories: 1,680
	Total Fat: 63 g	Total Fat: 66 g	Total Fat: 61 g
	Saturated Fat: 12 g	Saturated Fat: 19 g	Saturated Fat: 22 g
	Carbohydrate: 137 g	Carbohydrate: 141 g	Carbohydrate: 157 g
	Protein: 121 g	Protein: 135 g	Protein: 137 g
	Sodium: 1,234 mg	Sodium: 2,605 mg	Sodium: 1,869 mg
	Cholesterol: 346 mg	Cholesterol: 265 mg	Cholesterol: 201 mg
	Fiber: 31 g	Fiber: 26 g	Fiber: 37 g

• • •

"Fearfully." "Wonderfully." "Knit together." "Formed." "Created." These are just a few of the ways the Bible describes how God lovingly built us. Just imagine Him with a level as He designed our souls with integrity. Picture it as He wipes the dust from our rough edges, smoothing tempers and molding character. It's no wonder He chose to be a carpenter. We're a masterpiece that He signed with His blood and framed with a body. What a privilege it is to care for that work!

Day 4	Day 5	Day 6	Day 7
Calories: 1,626	Calories: 1,601	Calories: 1,616	Calories: 1,621
Total Fat: 56 g	Total Fat: 64 g	Total Fat: 66 g	Total Fat: 67 g
Saturated Fat: 8 g	Saturated Fat: 20 g	Saturated Fat: 20 g	Saturated Fat: 14 g
Carbohydrate: 154 g	Carbohydrate: 141 g	Carbohydrate: 153 g	Carbohydrate: 148 g
Protein: 134 g	Protein: 126 g	Protein: 116 g	Protein: 114 g
Sodium: 1,984 mg	Sodium: 1,288 mg	Sodium: 1,061 mg	Sodium: 2,569 mg
Cholesterol: 220 mg	Cholesterol: 266 mg	Cholesterol: 238 mg	Cholesterol: 514 mg
Fiber: 34 g	Fiber: 37 g	Fiber: 21 g	Fiber: 26 g

So when you think of creation as His handiwork, just look in the mirror. When you consider the *breadth* of His work, take a deep *breath* yourself. Let the scale's evidence and the slowly building godly confidence you feel be a stamp of approval upon week 3. After all, when He said, "It was very good," He was looking at you. What did He see? His image. Remember, you're His handiwork. How you fuel your body matters. See you in week 4, friends.

WEEK 3

How are you feeling this third week?

_____

_____

Any praises and successes that you're excited to write down?

_____

_____

Do you notice any physical changes—do your clothes fit better? Have you seen any results on the scale?

_____

_____

What about pitfalls and setbacks? What were they and could they have been avoided? What steps will you take this next week to avoid them?

_____

_____

How did the meal prep go? Did you skip any meals? Which ones? Did you prepare some meals in advance? Which ones? Did other members of your household enjoy some or all of the meals you prepared?

_____

_____

What was your favorite dinner?

_____

_____

Are you playing _your_ song of creation? Knowing that your life is an instrument designed to play in God's arrangement, how has the change in your eating pattern helped your enthusiasm to chime in?

_____

_____

Does the reality of a slimmer, healthier, and more active version of "you" help you want to live out loud?

_____

_____

Are you amazed at the kinds of results you're seeing and feeling?

_____

_____

Do you want to share with others for Whom as well as why you've made such incredible changes?

_____

_____

Are you spending quality time alone with God? Does your prayer time and Bible study equal in importance with your desire to lose weight or improve your health?

_____

_____

What measures do you need to take to ensure you're growing spiritually?

_____

_____

Are you keeping in touch with a trusted friend or family member to help hold you accountable in your spiritual and physical objectives? Do you hold them accountable as well?

_____

_____

COMMITMENT: I am so thankful for the progress I'm making. Old habits are losing their grip on me. I'm learning about what foods do to my body and what my body is able to do because of my new balanced meal plan. This week, I commit to the Lord, myself, and my family that I will _____ in week 4 in order to live a healthier, more active, and abundant life.

PRAYER: *Lord God, I love you and I thank you for another week to serve you with my health. I thank you for never leaving my side. During good times and bad times, you're in control. You never panic. Thank you for being my rock, my shelter, my healer. Help everything I do and say and everything I eat and the exercise I perform bring you honor and praise. In Jesus' name, amen.*

10

WEEK 4

MOVE WITH YOUR LIFE

Turn to any page in God's word and you'll find the countless biblical examples of people who had physical reactions to Jesus, either to be *near* Him or because they had just been *with* Him. It's simple, He just moves us! But there was one person who didn't move a muscle.

The criminal had just been given Heaven. Every sin of his wasted years had been forgiven, his name had just been written in the Lamb's book of life, and soon the angels would be teaching him to sing. And yet, despite this gift of grace and mercy, He didn't run to embrace Him. He didn't leap for joy, lift his hands in praise, or kneel in worship. Why? Well, he *couldn't* move. See, the nails were too deep, the pain was too great. If he could've climbed down from that cross, he probably would've demonstrated *physically* what his heart had experienced *spiritually*.

What about you? You may be eighteen or eighty, and Lord

knows this brief life is not about the body, but if you've been given Heaven, week 4 on the PrayFit Diet represents another opportunity to move, another chance to respond to what God has done, what He is doing, and what He will do through your new, abundant, health-filled life.

WEEK 4 SHOPPING LIST

Produce

Mango: 1 (A tangy fruit that is filled with craving-crushing fiber.)

Lime: 1

Pomegranate: 1

Pineapple: 1

Orange: 1

Grapefruit: 2

Apple: 1 (Don't let people tell you that you can't have fruit on a weight-loss diet. Apples, in particular, are loaded with fiber [5 grams] that helps you exercise dietary restraint. The fiber also improves digestion to help you better absorb other fat-fighting nutrients in the PrayFit Diet.)

Lemons: 1

Berries: 1 pint

Tomatoes: 3

Swiss chard: 1 bunch

Baby carrots: 1 bag

Mushrooms: ½ pound

Red bell pepper: 1 (These brightly colored, antioxidant-filled veggies add flavor and fiber to your plate and can be used to make healthy salsas.)

Cucumber: 1

Cilantro: 1 small bunch

Spinach: ½ pound

Broccoli: 2 large bunches

Leeks: 1

Fresh tarragon: 1 bunch

Sweet potatoes: 2

Zucchini: 1 large

Lettuce

Dairy and Eggs

Eggs: 1 dozen

Low-fat Swiss cheese: ¼ pound

Nonfat Greek yogurt: 1 cup

Shredded cheddar cheese: ¼ cup

Low-fat cottage cheese: 32 ounces

Low-fat pepper jack cheese: 2 ounces

Part-skim mozzarella cheese

Bakery

Ezekiel tortilla

Whole-wheat English muffin

Ezekiel bread

Corn tortillas (Contain about one third the calories of flour
tortillas.)

Meat, Deli, Seafood

Tilapia: ½ pound (Tilapia is light, firm, affordable, and easy to
cook. It's an example of a farmed fish that's actually a good
choice.)

Boneless, skinless chicken breast: 2½ pounds

Flank steak: ⅓ pound

Salmon: ⅓ pound

Pork tenderloin: ½ pound (On the whole, pork tenderloin has
less fat than chicken breast, making it a great, lower-calorie
protein choice.)

Grocery, Pantry

- Hot sauce
- Rolled oats
- Honey
- Almonds
- Cinnamon
- Balsamic vinegar
- Walnuts
- Bow-tie pasta
- Prepared pesto
- Green tea
- Chicken broth
- Canned artichoke hearts
- Natural peanut butter
- White beans (This fiber- and protein-heavy legume slows digestion down to a crawl, meaning fewer cravings later. It's also full of vitamins and minerals.)
- BBQ sauce
- Semisweet chocolate chips
- Minestrone soup
- Dijon mustard
- Jam
- Salsa

Frozen

- Mango chunks
- Edamame

WEEK 4 MEAL PLAN

Days 22–28	Day 1	Day 2	Day 3
Breakfast	Honey-Nut Oatmeal 1 tablespoon natural peanut butter Calories: 361 Total Fat: 18 g Saturated Fat: 3 g Carbohydrate: 44 g Protein: 11 g Sodium: 17 mg Cholesterol: 0 mg Fiber: 7 g	Tomato, Mushroom, and Swiss Omelet Calories: 318 Total Fat: 18 g Saturated Fat: 7 g Carbohydrate: 7 g Protein: 36 g Sodium: 487 mg Cholesterol: 392 mg Fiber: 1 g	Mango Green Tea Smoothie Calories: 305 Total Fat: 1 g Saturated Fat: 0 g Carbohydrate: 67 g Protein: 12 g Sodium: 63 mg Cholesterol: 7 mg Fiber: 5 g
Lunch	5 oz grilled chicken breast ½ cup cooked brown rice ½ cup white beans 2 cups chicken broth Calories: 542 Total Fat: 9 g Saturated Fat: 3 g Carbohydrate: 51 g Protein: 65 g Sodium: 259 mg Cholesterol: 120 mg Fiber: 7 g	Turkey Quesadilla (made with 2 Ezekiel tortillas, 2 oz deli turkey, ½ cup shredded cheddar cheese, BBQ sauce) Calories: 436 Total Fat: 11 g Saturated Fat: 1 g Carbohydrate: 59 g Protein: 27 g Sodium: 1,266 mg Cholesterol: 37 mg Fiber: 10	2½ cups low-sodium minestrone soup 1 piece part-skim string cheese Calories: 571 Total Fat: 33 g Saturated Fat: 8 g Carbohydrate: 63 g Protein: 35 g Sodium: 941 mg Cholesterol: 10 mg Fiber: 10 g

Day 4	Day 5	Day 6	Day 7
4 egg whites, scrambled with ¼ cup spinach and 1 slice low-fat pepper jack cheese 2 slices Ezekiel toast ½ grapefruit Calories: 337 Total Fat: 4 g Saturated Fat: 2 g Carbohydrate: 44 g Protein: 32 g Sodium: 650 mg Cholesterol: 6 mg Fiber: 9 g	1 whole-wheat English muffin 1 tablespoon natural peanut butter 1 cup raspberries or blueberries Calories: 309 Total Fat: 1 g Saturated Fat: 2 g Carbohydrate: 44 g Protein: 11 g Sodium: 226 mg Cholesterol: 0 mg Fiber: 12 g	Honey-Nut Oatmeal 1 hard-boiled egg Calories: 334 Total Fat: 14 g Saturated Fat: 3 g Carbohydrate: 42 g Protein: 13 g Sodium: 64 mg Cholesterol: 187 mg Fiber: 5 g	Mango Green Tea Smoothie Calories: 305 Total Fat: 1 g Saturated Fat: 0 g Carbohydrate: 67 g Protein: 12 g Sodium: 63 mg Cholesterol: 7 mg Fiber: 5 g
Spinach Salad with Walnuts and Pomegranate 4 oz grilled chicken breast Calories: 691 Total Fat: 37 g Saturated Fat: 8 g Carbohydrate: 20 g Protein: 70 g Sodium: 881 mg Cholesterol: 172 mg Fiber: 6 g	4 oz deli turkey or roast beef 1 slice Swiss cheese Dijon mustard Sliced tomato 2 slices Ezekiel bread Calories: 457 Total Fat: 14 g Saturated Fat: 8 g Carbohydrate: 36 g Protein: 36 g Sodium: 967 mg Cholesterol: 125 mg Fiber: 6 g	1 Ezekiel tortilla 3 tablespoons natural peanut butter 1 tablespoon jam Calories: 521 Total Fat: 29 g Saturated Fat: 5 g Carbohydrate: 47 g Protein: 17 g Sodium: 191 mg Cholesterol: 0 mg Fiber: 10 g	Spinach Salad with Walnuts and Pomegranate 4 oz grilled chicken breast Calories: 691 Total Fat: 37 g Saturated Fat: 8 g Carbohydrate: 20 g Protein: 70 g Sodium: 881 mg Cholesterol: 172 mg Fiber: 6 g

Days 22–28	Day 1	Day 2	Day 3
Snack	1 cup low-fat cottage cheese ½ cup chopped pineapple 10 baby carrots Calories: 239 Total Fat: 3 g Saturated Fat: 1 g Carbohydrate: 25 g Protein: 29 g Sodium: 996 mg Cholesterol: 9 mg Fiber: 4 g	1 cup steamed edamame 1 clementine or orange Calories: 189 Total Fat: 8 g Saturated Fat: 1 g Carbohydrate: 15 g Protein: 17 g Sodium: 9 mg Cholesterol: 0 mg Fiber: 8 g	½ cup low-fat cottage cheese ¼ cup almonds Calories: 287 Total Fat: 19 g Saturated Fat: 2 g Carbohydrate: 11 g Protein: 22 g Sodium: 459 mg Cholesterol: 5 mg Fiber: 4 g
Dinner	4 oz flank steak 1 baked sweet potato 2 cups steamed broccoli 1 tablespoon olive oil Calories: 493 Total Fat: 22 g Saturated Fat: 6 g Carbohydrate: 34 g Protein: 38 g Sodium: 176 mg Cholesterol: 88 mg Fiber: 8 g	Tilapia with Mango Salsa 2 cups cooked zucchini Calories: 543 Total Fat: 20 g Saturated Fat: 3 g Carbohydrate: 46 g Protein: 52 g Sodium: 274 mg Cholesterol: 113 mg Fiber: 9 g	6 oz grilled or roasted boneless, skinless chicken breast 2 cups cooked broccoli Lemon juice Chocolate Dipped Oranges Calories: 531 Total Fat: 19 g Saturated Fat: 7 g Carbohydrate: 33 g Protein: 59 g Sodium: 164 mg Cholesterol: 145 mg Fiber: 3 g

Day 4	Day 5	Day 6	Day 7
1 medium apple 1 tablespoon peanut or almond butter Calories: 200 Total Fat: 9 g Saturated Fat: 2 g Carbohydrate: 28 g Protein: 4 g Sodium: 17 mg Cholesterol: 0 mg Fiber: 6 g	1 grapefruit 1 hard-boiled egg Calories: 151 Total Fat: 6 g Saturated Fat: 2 g Carbohydrate: 19 g Protein: 8 g Sodium: 62 mg Cholesterol: 187 mg Fiber: 3 g	1 cup low-fat cottage cheese 10 baby carrots Calories: 198 Total Fat: 2 g Saturated Fat: 1 g Carbohydrate: 14 g Protein: 29 g Sodium: 996 mg Cholesterol: 9 mg Fiber: 3 g	1 cup nonfat Greek yogurt ½ cup chopped pineapple Calories: 161 Total Fat: 0 g Saturated Fat: 0 g Carbohydrate: 14 g Protein: 20 g Sodium: 86 mg Cholesterol: 0 mg Fiber: 1 g
5 oz roasted salmon 3 cups Swiss chard sautéed in 1 tablespoon olive oil and lemon juice 1 baked sweet potato Calories: 449 Total Fat: 12 g Saturated Fat: 2 g Carbohydrate: 46 g Protein: 42 g Sodium: 240 mg Cholesterol: 78 mg Fiber: 8 g	Chicken and Bow Ties Calories: 691 Total Fat: 32 g Saturated Fat: 7 g Carbohydrate: 54 g Protein: 49 g Sodium: 994 mg Cholesterol: 79 mg Fiber: 10 g	5 oz grilled pork tenderloin, thinly sliced 3 corn tortillas ⅓ cup salsa Shredded lettuce Hot sauce Calories: 550 Total Fat: 16 g Saturated Fat: 5 g Carbohydrate: 44 g Protein: 57 g Sodium: 894 mg Cholesterol: 160 mg Fiber: 6 g	Chicken Jerusalem Calories: 543 Total Fat: 18 g Saturated Fat: 3 g Carbohydrate: 26 g Protein: 61 g Sodium: 1,817 mg Cholesterol: 131 mg Fiber: 11 g

Days 22–28	Day 1	Day 2	Day 3
Totals for the Day	Calories: 1,636	Calories: 1,486	Calories: 1,694
	Total Fat: 52 g	Total Fat: 57 g	Total Fat: 71 g
	Saturated Fat: 12 g	Saturated Fat: 12 g	Saturated Fat: 17 g
	Carbohydrate: 154 g	Carbohydrate: 128 g	Carbohydrate: 149 g
	Protein: 142 g	Protein: 131 g	Protein: 127 g
	Sodium: 1,449 mg	Sodium: 2,037 mg	Sodium: 1,627 mg
	Cholesterol: 218 mg	Cholesterol: 543 mg	Cholesterol: 219 mg
	Fiber: 26 g	Fiber: 28 g	Fiber: 22 g

• • •

The story of the criminal from the beginning of our chapter reminds me of one of my personal journal entries:

On Sunday in church, I sat behind a man who was paralyzed from the neck down. It was interesting to me that when the choir director asked the congregation to stand and sing, you could feel the reluctance and see the slow-moving crowd rise to their feet. I thought, *I wonder how fast this sweet man would stand if he could.* The next song we sang was "Bless the Lord, oh my soul, and all that is within me, bless His Holy name." You know what? This man's voice was the loudest one around me. Plainly said, when we were asked to stand, he already was standing. Folks, life is not about the body, so if you have health and ability, use it as a means of praise. And believer, if you're called to stand and sing and you can, stand up and sing.

Friends, how many times have we asked God to move in our lives? I wonder if it even comes close to the number of times He's asked us to move *with* ours. Follow me through the day: the homeless beggar outside the supermarket; the lonely neighbor nobody ever seems to talk to; the teacher everybody gossips about. How many times a day does God ask us to move *with* our lives?

Day 4	Day 5	Day 6	Day 7
Calories: 1,677	Calories: 1,608	Calories: 1,602	Calories: 1,700
Total Fat: 61 g	Total Fat: 62 g	Total Fat: 62 g	Total Fat: 56 g
Saturated Fat: 14 g	Saturated Fat: 19 g	Saturated Fat: 14 g	Saturated Fat: 11 g
Carbohydrate: 138 g	Carbohydrate: 153 g	Carbohydrate: 147 g	Carbohydrate: 133 g
Protein: 148 g	Protein: 115 g	Protein: 116 g	Protein: 163 g
Sodium: 1,788 mg	Sodium: 2,249 mg	Sodium: 2,145 mg	Sodium: 2,847 mg
Cholesterol: 256 mg	Cholesterol: 391 mg	Cholesterol: 355 mg	Cholesterol: 310 mg
Fiber: 29 g	Fiber: 32 g	Fiber: 24 g	Fiber: 23 g

Same goes with our bodies. You may find yourself asking the Lord for the strength to stick with this new amazing plan. But friends, if you know Him, He's already made His move. The real question is whether the miracle He's done in your heart has reached your feet. I believe it has. I believe the end of week 4 represents more than a month of diligence and hard work: it represents a true commitment to lose weight for life and a ton of heart work. You're moving with your life in the right direction. All this food, all this knowledge, these choices, recipes, and calories? Mile markers of a life that's been moved. I'm so proud of you. Let's finish strong.

WEEK 4

How are you feeling this week?

_____

_____

Any praises and successes that you're excited to write down?

_____

_____

Do you notice any physical changes—do your clothes fit better? Have you seen any results on the scale?

_____

_____

What about pitfalls and setbacks? What were they and could they have been avoided? What steps will you take this next week to avoid them?

_____

_____

Now that you're well into the plan, write down some of the secrets, tactics, and techniques you've incorporated into your routine to keep you on track.

_____

_____

What was your favorite snack? Have you shared some of your meals or snacks with family and friends? How was their experience?

_____

_____

We discussed in the text how week 4 was a new opportunity to move for the cause of Christ. What did you do to move with your life?

_____

_____

Knowing God made you for a reason and a mission, how does it make you feel knowing that your health is helping you live that purpose to its fullest?

_____

_____

Are you closer to the Lord than you were before you started the PrayFit Diet?

_____

_____

How has your relationship with food helped mold your personal relationship with Jesus?

_____

_____

COMMITMENT: I am blessed. I know there are those less fortunate. I will never again take my health for granted. I want to move with my life and make a difference in the lives of others for as long as I can. This week, I commit to the Lord, myself, and my family that I will _____ in week 5 in order to live a healthier, more active, and abundant life.

PRAYER: *Lord, I love you. I know there is never a moment I don't need you. I can never earn your grace. Thank you for my life and the blessings you've given me. Help me to be a better steward of all you've bestowed upon me, and the things you've placed in my care, including my body. Let my life bring you praise. In Jesus' name, amen.*

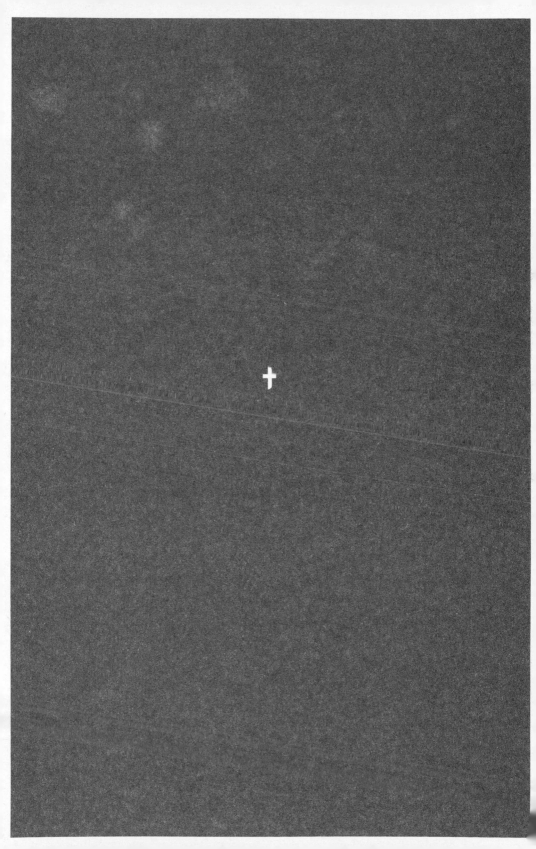

11

WEEK 5

As you start the last week of the PrayFit Diet, I thought I'd let Paul pay us another visit. The Apostle Paul knew that athletes live, eat, and sleep their sport. He understood the rigors, the devotion, the sacrifices, and the quest to be the one to win. Paul wrote in the Bible, "I discipline my body like an athlete, training it to do what it should." In fact, to encourage us in our spiritual lives, Paul regularly talked about runners and the devotion required to succeed in their sport, reminding us of our need to be steadfast in our days.

But unlike the runner who trains *for* a race, we train *during* one. So as you embark on week 5 of the PrayFit Diet, I want you to pay special attention to the second half of the verse I mentioned above. Notice what he said: "training [a process] it [the body] to do [to act, proceed] what it should [the right thing]."

Paul wants us to train our eyes to notice the lonely, our ears to hear the helpless. He wants to train us to deny the flesh. We're to run to Christ, run away from sin, run to those in need, and do it all the time.

And he knew that for us to do that, we have to live, eat, and sleep the Word of God. He also knew that we need our health—these bodies—functioning properly to accomplish our purpose. The meal plans, recipes, and calorie counts that you'll enjoy during week 5 serve to further establish your physical ability to do what you were meant to do: healthier, slimmer, wiser, stronger.

So as you start your last week of the PrayFit Diet, let the words of Paul invigorate you. You've shown the discipline of an athlete when it comes to healthier food and habits. You're training your body like an athlete so you can do what you should. You're in great company; the best that ever was. Ready, set, go . . .

WEEK 5 SHOPPING LIST

Produce

Apples: 3

Banana: 1

Lemons: 3

Orange: 1

Grapefruit: 1

Berries: 1 pint

Clementine: 1 (A sweet, easy-to-peel, portable fruit containing fiber and immune-boosting vitamin C.)

Fresh rosemary: 1 bunch

Green cabbage: 1 head

Carrots: 1

Lettuce: 1 head

Baby spinach: 8 cups

Mixed greens: 1 package (4 cups)

Tomatoes: 1

Mushrooms: ¼ pound

Beets: 2

Garlic: 1 head

Yellow onion: 1

Green beans: ½ pound (2 cups)

Bell pepper: 1

Zucchini: 1 large

Spaghetti squash (Contains slow-digesting carbs for energy and is saturated with antioxidants.)

Dairy and Eggs

2% flavored Greek yogurt: 2.5 cups

Nonfat Greek yogurt: 8 ounces

Nonfat vanilla Greek yogurt: 16 ounces

Eggs: 1 dozen

Part-skim string cheese: 1 small package

Low-fat Swiss cheese: 2 ounces

Low-fat cheddar cheese: 2 ounces

Crumbled goat cheese: 2 ounces (Goat cheese offers a hearty helping of calcium. Diets rich in calcium have proven to help the body burn fat more effectively after meals.)

Skim milk

Crumbled feta cheese: ¼ cup

Bakery

Ezekiel or whole-wheat tortilla

Ezekiel bread

Corn tortillas

Meat, Deli, Seafood

Boneless pork chops: ½ pound

Ground turkey breast: 1½ pounds

Shrimp: ¾ pound (Low in calories, high in protein, shrimp is a great addition to any weight-management program.)

Deli turkey: ⅓ pound

Salmon: ½ pound

Boneless, skinless chicken breast: ½ pound

Flank steak: ⅓ pound

Grocery, Pantry

Celery salt

Balsamic vinegar

Honey

Walnuts

Dijon mustard

Canned tuna

Whole-grain cereal

Rolled oats

Sliced almonds

Shredded sweetened coconut

Shredded unsweetened coconut

Maple syrup

Dried apricots

Dried oregano

Dried ground fennel

Crushed tomatoes

Dried cranberries (Fiber- and iron-dense, these are a great "anywhere" snack.)

Salsa

Chili powder (Use chili powder for roasting meat or fish. It provides *big* flavor with few calories.)

Hot sauce (Hot sauce can instantly jazz up your favorite protein dish. It also contains capsaicin, a powerful compound known for its ability to trigger fat loss. Go easy, though, it is heavy in sodium.)

Frozen

Edamame: 1 bag

WEEK 5 MEAL PLAN

Days 29–33	Day 1	Day 2	Day 3
Breakfast	Tomato, Mushroom, and Swiss Omelet 1 slice Ezekiel bread Calories: 398 Total Fat: 18 g Saturated Fat: 8 g Carbohydrate: 22 g Protein: 40 g Sodium: 567 mg Cholesterol: 392 mg Fiber: 4 g	½ cup Coconut-Apricot Granola 1½ cups nonfat Greek vanilla yogurt Calories: 399 Total Fat: 9 g Saturated Fat: 3 g Carbohydrate: 46 g Protein: 35 g Sodium: 179 mg Cholesterol: 0 mg Fiber: 4 g	Breakfast Salad Calories: 501 Total Fat: 29 g Saturated Fat: 10 g Carbohydrate: 63 g Protein: 8 g Sodium: 9 mg Cholesterol: 0 mg Fiber: 14 g
Lunch	Tuna and Olive Wrap ½ cup edamame Calories: 420 Total Fat: 17 g Saturated Fat: 1 g Carbohydrate: 37 g Protein: 36 g Sodium: 1,099 mg Cholesterol: 38 mg Fiber: 9 g	Roasted Beet Salad 3 oz grilled shrimp Calories: 489 Total Fat: 26 g Saturated Fat: 9 g Carbohydrate: 26 g Protein: 39 g Sodium: 441 mg Cholesterol: 95 mg Fiber: 8 g	Turkey wrap (1 Ezekiel tortilla, 3 oz deli turkey, 1 slice low-fat cheddar cheese, Dijon mustard, vegetables such as grated carrots, sliced cucumber, or bell peppers) Calories: 344 Total Fat: 9 g Saturated Fat: 1 g Carbohydrate: 37 g Protein: 29 g Sodium: 915 mg Cholesterol: 68 mg Fiber: 6 g

Day 4	Day 5
2 cups whole-grain cereal 1 cup milk or soy milk ½ cup berries	¾ cup Coconut-Apricot Granola 1 cup skim milk 1 clementine
Calories: 391 Total Fat: 5 g Saturated Fat: 0 g Carbohydrate: 44 g Protein: 11 g Sodium: 132 mg Cholesterol: 5 mg Fiber: 2 g	Calories: 485 Total Fat: 16 g Saturated Fat: 4 g Carbohydrate: 74 g Protein: 17 g Sodium: 180 mg Cholesterol: 5 mg Fiber: 8 g
4 oz grilled chicken or turkey breast 1 cup chopped tomato 3 cups mixed greens ¼ cup crumbled feta cheese 1 tablespoon olive oil + balsamic vinegar	Roasted Beet Salad 3 oz grilled chicken or shrimp
Calories: 471 Total Fat: 27 g Saturated Fat: 8 g Carbohydrate: 25 g Protein: 50 g Sodium: 635 mg Cholesterol: 107 mg Fiber: 14 g	Calories: 489 Total Fat: 26 g Saturated Fat: 9 g Carbohydrate: 26 g Protein: 39 g Sodium: 441 mg Cholesterol: 95 mg Fiber: 8 g

Days 29–33	Day 1	Day 2	Day 3
Snack	¼ cup dried cranberries 1 apple Calories: 200 Total Fat: 0 g Saturated Fat: 0 g Carbohydrate: 51 g Protein: 0 g Sodium: 2 mg Cholesterol: 0 mg Fiber: 6 g	2 oz deli turkey 1 banana Calories: 169 Total Fat: 2 g Saturated Fat: 0 g Carbohydrate: 31 g Protein: 9 g Sodium: 682 mg Cholesterol: 31 mg Fiber: 3 g	2 hard-boiled eggs Calories: 155 Total Fat: 11 g Saturated Fat: 3 g Carbohydrate: 1 g Protein: 13 g Sodium: 124 mg Cholesterol: 373 mg Fiber: 0 g
Dinner	5 oz turkey burger 2 cups steamed green beans Frozen Greek Yogurt Calories: 501 Total Fat: 20 g Saturated Fat: 5 g Carbohydrate: 25 g Protein: 42 g Sodium: 110 mg Cholesterol: 120 mg Fiber: 6 g	6 oz salmon, roasted with 1 tablespoon olive oil and chili powder 3 corn tortillas ½ cup salsa Shredded lettuce Hot sauce Calories: 564 Total Fat: 23 g Saturated Fat: 4 g Carbohydrate: 44 g Protein: 46 g Sodium: 884 mg Cholesterol: 94 mg Fiber: 6 g	Pork Chops with Apple Slaw Calories: 542 Total Fat: 19 g Saturated Fat: 1 g Carbohydrate: 43 g Protein: 52 g Sodium: 1,907 mg Cholesterol: 156 mg Fiber: 8 g

Day 4	Day 5
1 medium apple 1 piece part-skim string cheese	¼ cup walnuts 2 tablespoons dried cranberries
Calories: 185 Total Fat: 6 g Saturated Fat: 4 g Carbohydrate: 26 g Protein: 9 g Sodium: 212 mg Cholesterol: 20 mg Fiber: 4 g	Calories: 249 Total Fat: 20 g Saturated Fat: 2 g Carbohydrate: 17 g Protein: 5 g Sodium: 1 mg Cholesterol: 0 mg Fiber: 3 g
5 oz grilled/ broiled flank steak 2 cups cooked zucchini 1 tablespoon olive oil, lemon juice, and crushed garlic	Turkey Meat Sauce 2 cups cooked spaghetti squash 2 cups baby spinach 1 tablespoon olive oil + balsamic vinegar
Calories: 490 Total Fat: 28 g Saturated Fat: 7 g Carbohydrate: 10 g Protein: 52 g Sodium: 108 mg Cholesterol: 133 mg Fiber: 4 g	Calories: 507 Total Fat: 22 g Saturated Fat: 3 g Carbohydrate: 43 g Protein: 37 g Sodium: 603 mg Cholesterol: 71 mg Fiber: 12 g

Days 29–33	Day 1	Day 2	Day 3
Totals for the Day	Calories: 1,519	Calories: 1,621	Calories: 1,542
	Total Fat: 56 g	Total Fat: 60 g	Total Fat: 68 g
	Saturated Fat: 14 g	Saturated Fat: 16 g	Saturated Fat: 16 g
	Carbohydrate: 136 g	Carbohydrate: 148 g	Carbohydrate: 144 g
	Protein: 118 g	Protein: 129 g	Protein: 101 g
	Sodium: 1,778 mg	Sodium: 2,186 mg	Sodium: 2,955 mg
	Cholesterol: 550 mg	Cholesterol: 220 mg	Cholesterol: 597 mg
	Fiber: 25 g	Fiber: 22 g	Fiber: 28 g

• • •

Have you ever witnessed a false start at a track meet? They're tough to watch. On some of sports' grandest stages, many of track and field's top athletes stumble right out of the blocks or, worse, jump the gun—disqualification from a race you've trained your entire life for is arguably one of the roughest moments to witness.

If anyone in the Bible could attest to false starts and rough beginnings, it was Paul. Yes indeed. One of Christianity's most zealous enemies, Paul approved of the stoning of Stephen (Acts 7:58). The very same man whose hands wrote of godly discipline was once *merciless*. But a face-to-face with the Author of Mercy Himself changed all that. Following his conversion, Paul carried out his mission in the face of mental and physical hardship the likes of which we have never imagined. His tireless preaching and unparalleled endurance have inspired countless missionaries for two thousand years, not to mention me as I'm typing this sentence.

But despite his false start, Paul said, "I discipline my body like an athlete, training it to do what it should. So that after I have preached to others I myself will not be disqualified." Why did he discipline himself like an athlete and train himself to do the right thing? Simple. So that he would be seen running the same race in the same way that he urged us to run. False starts, stumbles,

Day 4	Day 5
Calories: 1,537	Calories: 1,730
Total Fat: 66 g	Total Fat: 84 g
Saturated Fat: 20 g	Saturated Fat: 19 g
Carbohydrate: 105 g	Carbohydrate: 158 g
Protein: 112 g	Protein: 99 g
Sodium: 1,087 mg	Sodium: 1,280 mg
Cholesterol: 265 mg	Cholesterol: 171 mg
Fiber: 24 g	Fiber: 30 g

and tumbles are no match for the grace of God, but they're tough to witness and tough on our witness. Truly, Paul pleaded for physical and spiritual discipline not in order to earn grace but because of the gift of it. He finished strong. Oh for grace, may we all do the same.

Maybe "false start" is a good way to describe the way you used to feel about your health. Perhaps you jumped the gun or ignored what you knew down deep inside was the right way to live, move, and eat. But after finishing week 5 of the PrayFit Diet, your false start is the last thing on your mind. Turning your newly trained mind and heart toward protein, fats, and carbs is a new beginning. You now see the end of week 5 as the starting block for an entirely new way of living, of feeling, of eating. Finally, a balanced approach like your body always wanted, your life always needed, your heart always strived for, and the Lord always intended. Grace, perspective, balance, abundance, and discipline: sounds an awful lot like an athlete.

WEEK 5

Well? How amazing does it feel to complete the five-week journey?

_____

_____

Any praises and successes that you're excited to write down?

_____

_____

How about the actual physical changes? If losing weight was your goal at the start, how many pounds did you lose? Do your clothes fit better?

_____

_____

What is your energy level now compared to the start of the plan? On a scale of 1 to 10, with 10 being high, how thrilled are you to be fitter and healthier?

_____

_____

On the flip side, what about pitfalls and setbacks? Did the last week present any insurmountable challenges? What will you do next week to make sure you correct and modify your routine to ensure excellence?

_____

_____

Next week? That's right, just because you've completed the plan doesn't mean it ends. At least it doesn't have to. You can now embark on the plan again, make changes, switch things up. The number of combinations of meals and foods is innumerable. You now have the 33 percent balance. You never have to leave this way of eating. If you love the balance, you can assume the PrayFit Diet for the rest of your life.

_____

_____

What was your favorite week? What foods or recipes are your absolute favorites? Have you shared some of them with family and friends? How was their experience?

_____

_____

How has the Apostle Paul and the way he disciplined his body helped you discipline your own?

_____

_____

Does knowing that even the founders of our faith used physical metaphors and endured physical struggle for the cause of Christ ignite the fire inside your heart?

_____

_____

We know that Paul disciplined his body and trained it to do what it should. What have you learned that you're able to do for others in your community, church, or home because of your renewed health?

_____

_____

Are you at a point in your health and life where you want to try a new activity? Maybe train for a 5K or even a marathon? Perhaps you want to pick up an old activity that you've been reluctant or unable to enjoy? What dream do you have that only your now renovated outlook and body can attempt? When you write it down, say (out loud) "Amen."

_____

_____

Who do you know that needs this book? Who do you love that needs a renewed perspective about the body? Write the name or names of those with whom you plan to share the PrayFit Diet. Jot them down. Say a prayer for them. Now act. Don't wait. When you do, remember that God doesn't need your health to get His message around the world, but you do. And now your health is restored in many ways, physically, emotionally, intellectually, and spiritually. It just might be time for you to help someone else.

_____

_____

COMMITMENT: What can I say? With God's help and by His grace, I did it. I finished the PrayFit Diet. I'm transformed from the inside out. I'm closer to the Lord in my heart and I've gained perspective about the biblical view of health. I've also regained my health. I've lost weight. I'm stronger, fitter, faster, healthier, better at home, at work, and at play. This week, I will share with someone I know and love about the importance of stewardship. And finally, I commit to the Lord, myself, and my family that I will _____ in order to live a healthier, more active, and abundant life as long as I live.

PRAYER: *Lord, thank you. I love you first and foremost for living in my heart. Thank you for securing my future, and I praise you for helping me live happier, healthier, and more abundant today. I pray that my life reflects the sacrifice you made to set me free forever. I pray that I treat my body and the food with which I sustain it with reverence. I am nothing without you, and I need my health to best serve you. I pray I never take my health for granted, but daily give you thanks and praise for each breath. In Jesus' name, amen.*

12

PRAYFIT
DIET RECIPES

"They all ate and were satisfied."

—MARK 6:42

The feeding of the five thousand is an amazing miracle moment, but when the crowds grew hungry, can't you just see the disciples on their tiptoes counting heads? I wonder what number they reached before they realized they were outnumbered? But just to be sure, they decided to count inventory of the basket. *"Two, three, four . . . nope, we're sure of it. Five loaves, two fish."*

If you're like me, depending on the day, you've been both the worried disciple and the hungry crowd. In either case, the only one we can ever count on is the only one *not* counting. But some days, I feel like the young boy in the story, don't you? Imagine him for a second. Little did he know that when his mom packed his bag that morning, he would *literally* hand it to God.

And while we don't hear the disciples say, *"Thanks, kid!"* or *"Glad you didn't come empty-handed, son,"* I like to imagine that after he got squeezed between the disciples and pushed to the back of the crowd, he found a nice spot on the hill with a good view. Grinning, he put his chin in his hands and watched God make a miracle out of his lunch.

We don't know what the next thirty-three days have in store, but we do know what we bring to each day, spiritually and physically. (I'm hoping these recipes help you "bring it.") And while you may not get applause for the changes you're making to your daily eating patterns, make sure to stick around to watch God do what only He can do with your life, and save me a seat. Because like our verse says, "They all ate." Even the little boy. You never know, maybe the boy grinned with his mouth full, and maybe Jesus Himself brought the little guy his meal. I'm not sure, but what we do know for certain is that our work *never* goes unnoticed (at least, not by the one who *doesn't count*).

Now, who's ready to go to work on some recipes?

As much as we'd all love to have a *Top Chef* contestant in our kitchen catering to our every dietary whim, there's a lot to be said for learning how to prepare healthy, great-tasting food on our own. The good news is that it's not as difficult as you might think. With just the shopping lists provided—you are, of course, welcome to add other nutrient-dense foods to your cart—you can use this list of recipes to create wholesome meals in minutes on your own, no sous-chef required.

The brilliance of the PrayFit Diet is in its simplicity. Complex carbs, lean proteins, and healthy fats—33 percent of your day's calories from each. Here we have provided creative, tasty ways to put these macronutrients together, every day, meal after health-filled meal. After just a few days, you'll have a very strong idea of how to plate perfectly proportioned meals with little to no guess-work. You'll also have a few extra recipes that you can dish up for friends and family.

Breakfasts

Honey-Nut Oatmeal
Serves 1

½ cup rolled oats
Water
2 teaspoons honey
2 tablespoons chopped almonds
Pinch cinnamon

Prepare oats according to package directions. Top with honey, al-monds, and cinnamon.

THE 33 DIFFERENCE: The dry rolled oats provide a great source of slow-digesting complex carbs for long-lasting energy. Honey gives you a quick jolt of healthy sugars to replenish fuel stores after your overnight fast. Almonds add great taste and texture to the oatmeal while providing quality fats to further slow digestion, and the cinnamon helps to stabilize blood sugar.

Breakfast Salad
Serves 1

2 cups orange and grapefruit segments
1 apple, sliced
¼ cup chopped walnuts
1 tablespoon unsweetened shredded coconut

Combine ingredients in a medium bowl; toss and serve.

THE 33 DIFFERENCE: Grapefruit is known for its ability to help your body burn more body fat, while the apples and oranges provide healthy fiber for sustained energy. Walnuts are a great source of healthy fats and antioxidants.

Mango Green Tea Smoothie
Serves 1

2 cups frozen mango chunks
½ cup nonfat Greek yogurt
1 cup brewed green tea
2 teaspoons honey

Place all ingredients into a blender. Blend until smooth.

THE 33 DIFFERENCE: Protein, fat, and carbs in fantastic proportions with a fat-fighting kick. The addition of green tea to this recipe provides EGCG, or epigallocatechin gallate, a powerful compound that inhibits the breakdown of norepinephrine, the neurohormone that revs up the metabolism. This smoothie helps you start your day the way you should: rebuilding muscle, fueling your day, and energizing you for hours.

Coconut-Apricot Granola
Makes about 4½ cups

Nonstick cooking spray
½ cups rolled oats
½ cup sliced almonds
½ cup shredded sweetened coconut
¼ teaspoon kosher salt
⅓ cup maple syrup or agave nectar
1 tablespoon canola oil
1 cup dried apricots, diced

Preheat oven to 300 degrees. Spray a large baking sheet with non-stick spray. In a large bowl combine oats, almonds, coconut, salt, maple syrup, and canola oil. Toss well and spread on prepared baking sheet in an even layer. Bake, stirring occasionally, until golden brown, about 15 to 20 minutes. Remove from oven. Once cool, mix in dried apricots. Store in an airtight container.

THE 33 DIFFERENCE: This recipe succeeds where sugary cereals fail by providing you long-lasting energy at a time when you need it the most. A hearty serving of oats will help you feel fuller longer and make you less likely to nosh on no-no foods at midmorning. The addition of shredded coconut and dried apricots adds vitamins and additional fiber to the mix. And that's before you add the milk!

Tomato, Mushroom, and Swiss Omelet
Serves 1

2 eggs
2 egg whites
1 tablespoon water
Salt and pepper to taste
½ cup chopped tomatoes
½ cup sliced mushrooms
Nonstick cooking spray
2 slices low-fat Swiss cheese

Heat a nonstick skillet over medium heat. Combine egg, egg whites, and water in a bowl, season with salt and pepper, and whisk well. Add tomatoes and mushrooms to egg mixture. Spray skillet with cooking spray. Add egg mixture and cook for 3 to 4 minutes until eggs begin to set. Using a spatula, gently pull in the sides of the omelet to let the uncooked egg run to the edges of the pan. Add cheese and gently fold in half. Allow to cook for 2 more minutes or until cheese is melted.

THE 33 DIFFERENCE: As you sleep, your body feasts on stored carbohydrates for energy. And once those stores are depleted, it can go on the hunt for additional energy. This can sometimes mean that it will take amino acids from muscles to convert into sugars for use. That's why it's important to get a healthy helping of protein as soon as you can get it in the morning. Eggs, as you learned in Chapter 4, are a great way to load up on protein and stave off midmorning cravings. The Swiss cheese adds a tasty upgrade to the omelet, while the mushrooms give you an immunity boost, as well as more B vitamins.

Lunches

Spinach Salad with Walnuts and Pomegranate
Serves 1

1 tablespoon extra-virgin olive oil
2 teaspoons balsamic vinegar or pomegranate juice
Salt and pepper
3 cups baby spinach
2 tablespoons chopped walnuts
1 cup diced cucumber
¼ cup pomegranate seeds
Protein add-on suggestions: grilled chicken, hard-boiled
    egg, cooked shrimp, broiled steak

In a medium bowl, whisk olive oil and vinegar. Season with salt and pepper. Add remaining ingredients to bowl and toss to coat with dressing.

THE 33 DIFFERENCE: Baby spinach happens to be one of the healthiest foods you can eat. It is also a tastier alternative for those who are bored with iceberg and romaine-based salads. High in healthy fat content due to the walnuts and olive oil, and loaded with fiber from the pomegranate, this salad can also be easily upgraded to include more protein.

Tuna and Olive Wrap
Serves 1

3 ounces canned tuna (water-packed)
¼ cup chopped olives (Kalamata or Nicoise recommended)
1 tablespoon nonfat Greek yogurt
1 whole-wheat tortilla
Mixed greens

In a small bowl combine tuna, olives, and yogurt, and mix well with fork. Place tuna mixture in tortilla and top with greens. Roll up and serve.

THE 33 DIFFERENCE: Midday, it's important to stay on the protein train. This tuna-based recipe is bolstered by protein-dense Greek yogurt and held together by a low-calorie whole-wheat tortilla. Chopped olives also give you some heart-healthy fats.

Vegetable Pizza
Serves 1

4 ounces whole-wheat pizza dough
Olive oil
½ cup chopped fresh tomato or prepared tomato sauce

1 cup fresh vegetables (suggestions: olives, bell pepper, mushrooms, kale, beet greens)

1 ounce shredded provolone cheese

2 ounces shredded part-skim mozzarella cheese

Fresh basil for garnish

Preheat oven to 450 degrees. Roll out pizza dough and transfer to a baking sheet that has been drizzled with olive oil. Top with sauce, vegetables, and cheese. Bake for 12 to 15 minutes until cheese is bubbly and crust is crispy. Garnish with fresh basil.

THE 33 DIFFERENCE: Pizza gets a bad rap. It doesn't have to be a greasy, indulgent, off-the-wagon treat reserved for date nights and birthday parties. When constructed with the right ingredients, it can be just as healthy as anything else in your diet. Not surprisingly, it comes down to balance, which is easy when you're making your own. Using a whole-wheat crust as your foundation, you are already at an advantage over your local delivery brand, because it won't impact your blood sugar in the same way as white-flour crusts. The sauce—made from veggies—actually has lycopene, which battles cancer and heart disease. The addition of cheese provides calcium and protein. Naturally, the 4-ounce serving represents a more sensible dose than you might be accustomed to, but the whole-wheat crust will also be more filling than your usual delivery pie.

Roasted Beet Salad
Serves 1

1 medium beet, diced

2 tablespoons olive oil, divided

Salt and pepper to taste

2 tablespoons freshly squeezed orange juice

3 cups baby spinach

½ cup shredded carrot

1 ounce goat cheese, crumbled

Preheat oven to 450 degrees. Place beets on a baking sheet. Drizzle with 1 tablespoon oil and season with salt and pepper. Roast for 10 to 15 minutes or until tender. In a bowl, whisk orange juice and olive oil, season with salt and pepper. Add spinach, carrots, and roasted beets to the bowl, toss to coat with dressing. Top with goat cheese and enjoy.

THE 33 DIFFERENCE: This sweet-tasting recipe will give you slow-burning carbs, healthy unsaturated fat, and, when paired with salmon or chicken, gives you everything you need for a balanced meal.

Dinners

Chicken Pesto and Bow Ties
Serves 1

2 ounces whole-grain bow-tie pasta (such as Barilla Plus)

1 tablespoon olive oil

5 ounces boneless, skinless chicken breast, cut into strips

¼ teaspoon kosher salt and black pepper to taste

1 tablespoon prepared pesto sauce

½ cup chopped fresh tomato

2 cups green vegetables (such as broccoli and zucchini)

2 tablespoons grated Parmesan cheese

Cook pasta according to package directions, reserving ½ cup of the cooking liquid. While pasta is cooking, heat oil in a large skillet over medium heat. Add chicken, season with salt and pepper, and cook for 3 to 4 minutes. Add pesto and vegetables and continue to cook for an additional 5 to 6 minutes, until chicken is cooked through. If mixture seems dry, add a small amount of the reserved pasta cooking liquid. Serve topped with grated Parmesan.

THE 33 DIFFERENCE: The PrayFit Diet isn't big on carbs, but we certainly didn't skimp on them. And in the realm of highly anticipated meals over the course of the next thirty-three days, this one probably ranks near the top. Pasta isn't necessarily an enemy for those trying to lose weight. In fact, when consumed with protein, the carbs from pasta are digested more slowly. And when the pasta is whole-grain, things slow down even more. The key is keeping your portion size to 2 ounces, along with your 5 ounces of chicken.

Pork Chops with Apple Slaw
Serves 1

8 ounces bone-in pork chops (about 1½ inches thick)
2 teaspoons olive oil
2 teaspoons chopped fresh rosemary
Salt and pepper

Apple Slaw
½ cup shredded green cabbage
1 green apple, grated
1 medium carrot, grated
1 teaspoon honey
Juice of ½ lemon
Pinch celery salt

Place pork chops in a resealable bag with oil, rosemary, salt, and pepper. Marinate for 30 minutes in the refrigerator.

For the slaw, place all ingredients in a medium bowl and toss well. Set aside.

Preheat grill or heavy-bottomed nonstick skillet over medium-high heat. Cook pork chops for about 5 minutes per side or until cooked through. Serve pork chop topped with slaw.

THE 33 DIFFERENCE: Sure, pork chops are the other white meat but that doesn't mean they have to be bland. This protein-heavy recipe is a vibrant combination of key ingredients that aid in fat loss and overall health. The apple slaw gives you a crunchy, sweet accompaniment that will make this one of your favorite repeat recipes long after these thirty-three days are over.

Chicken Jerusalem
Serves 1

1 tablespoon olive oil
½ pound boneless, skinless chicken breast, cut into strips
¼ teaspoon kosher salt and black pepper
½ cup sliced leeks (white and pale green parts only)
1 cup sliced mushrooms
1 cup chopped canned artichoke hearts, drained well
¼ cup white wine or chicken broth
2 tablespoons 2% Greek yogurt
1 tablespoon chopped fresh tarragon
Parmesan cheese for topping (optional)

Heat oil in a large skillet. Add chicken, season with salt and pepper, and cook for 2 to 3 minutes per side. Add leeks, mushrooms, artichoke hearts, and wine or broth to the pan and cook for an additional 6 to 8 minutes, or until chicken is cooked through. Add Greek yogurt and mix to combine. Garnish with fresh tarragon and Parmesan cheese, if using, and serve.

THE 33 DIFFERENCE: This favorite made the menu for two reasons. First of all, it tastes amazing. Second, it is a low-fat, low-carb, high-protein dinner that stores and reheats well. Though there are a few variations of this recipe floating around, this one represents the healthiest incarnation available without sacrificing flavor.

Gazpacho
Makes 2 servings

1 medium English cucumber
1 pound fresh tomatoes, roughly chopped (about 3 cups)
¼ cup low-sodium tomato juice
1 teaspoon red wine vinegar
1 tablespoon extra-virgin olive oil
1 medium bell pepper
2 tablespoons chopped fresh basil
Kosher salt
Freshly ground black pepper

Finely chop cucumber and set half aside. Place remaining cucumber, tomatoes, tomato juice, vinegar, olive oil, bell pepper, and basil in a food processor; season with ¾ teaspoon salt and pepper to taste. Pulse until well combined but not completely pureed. Transfer mixture to large bowl. Cover with plastic wrap and place in the refrigerator to chill for at least 2 hours. Serve chilled, topped with chopped cucumber.

THE 33 DIFFERENCE: Best served alongside a healthy protein, the PrayFit Diet gazpacho is a zesty, vitamin-rich recipe that can be enjoyed anytime. It is filled with healthy fat and fiber, making it a fantastic ally in your weight-loss efforts. The carotenoids in gazpacho may also help prevent some cancers and bolster eye health.

Turkey Meat Sauce

Makes 1 quart

2 tablespoons olive oil

1 cup chopped onion

2 cloves minced garlic

Kosher salt and freshly ground black pepper

2 teaspoons dried oregano

½ teaspoon dried ground fennel

1 pound ground turkey breast

1 can (28 ounces) crushed tomatoes

½ cup water

Red pepper flakes (optional)

Heat oil in a large skillet. Add onions and garlic; season with salt and pepper, and cook for 5 minutes. Add oregano, fennel, and turkey and season with an additional ¼ teaspoon of salt. Cook until turkey is browned. Add tomatoes and water; bring to a simmer, reduce heat, and cook for an additional 30 minutes. Season with red pepper flakes, if using, before serving.

THE 33 DIFFERENCE: Everyone appreciates a hearty meat sauce, but making it with red meat every time means more calories and saturated fat. Making the easy swap to ground turkey will provide you all the same flavor and texture but fewer calories and fat, without sacrificing in the protein department. Use this sauce to top an Ezekiel tortilla or a whole-wheat mini pizza crust to get your Italian fix . . . only healthier.

Tilapia with Mango Salsa
Serves 1

1 mango, peeled and diced
½ cup chopped red bell pepper
½ cup chopped cucumber
Juice of ½ lime
1 tablespoon chopped fresh cilantro
Salt
Hot sauce
8 ounces tilapia
1 tablespoon canola oil

For the salsa, combine mango, pepper, cucumber, lime juice, and cilantro. Season with salt and a few dashes of hot sauce, if desired; set aside.

Season tilapia with canola oil, salt, and hot sauce. Cook fish in a nonstick skillet or grill for 3 to 4 minutes per side or until completely cooked through. Serve topped with salsa.

THE 33 DIFFERENCE: Tilapia is a healthy, protein-loaded mainstay on the PrayFit Diet, and there are a number of ways you can prepare it. But after you try this recipe, you may be more of the "if it ain't broke, don't fix it" persuasion. By combining mango, bell pepper, cucumber, lime, and cilantro, you get a flavor explosion that jazzes up an already amazing source of protein and healthy dietary fat.

Snacks and Sides

Hummus
Makes 2 cups

1 can (15 ounces) chickpeas
1 tablespoon sesame tahini

¼ cup extra-virgin olive oil

Juice of ½ lemon

¼ teaspoon kosher salt

¼ teaspoon smoked paprika, or more to taste

Rinse and drain chickpeas. Combine ingredients in a food processor and pulse until smooth.

THE 33 DIFFERENCE: One of the keys to maintaining steady weight loss is to eat more of the right foods throughout the day. The times in between meals is what usually gets people into trouble. But if you have quick access to a healthy snack that also tastes good, you will have few excuses left for round-the-clock discipline. Hummus, which contains protein-heavy chickpeas, can be taken to work, the gym, or school in plastic containers and used as a dip for carrots, celery, Ezekiel bread, and more.

Frozen Greek Yogurt
Serves 1

¼ cup water

2½ cups 2% flavored Greek yogurt

Combine water and yogurt in a large bowl and whisk well. Transfer to an ice cream machine and mix according to manufacturer's directions. Serve immediately or place in a freezer-safe container for up to one week.

THE 33 DIFFERENCE: Slow-burning carbs and protein—a winning combination for fat loss—is the DNA of Greek yogurt. But you don't have to have it out of the container each time. You can freeze it to give it an ice-cream-like texture for a great after-dinner treat or a chilled midday snack.

Chocolate-Dipped Oranges
Serves 2

¼ cup semisweet chocolate chips
1 medium orange

Melt chocolate chips in a microwave-safe bowl. Peel orange and separate into segments. Dip orange segments into melted chocolate, transfer to a plate, and let the chocolate set. (For quicker setting, place chocolate-dipped oranges in the refrigerator for 10 minutes.)

THE 33 DIFFERENCE: Balance, not deprivation. But where are the treats, you ask? Well, you won't find cookies or cupcakes in these pages, but this easy-to-make treat—which is great to share with kids—allows you to get your fix of sweets without derailing your progress. Oranges, as you know, are rich in immune-boosting vitamin C and fiber to fill you up fast. Surprisingly, semisweet chocolate contains less fat and more antioxidants than milk chocolate. So eat up!

CONCLUSION

Jesus ate perfectly. Do you find that amazing? Whether during a hearty celebration meal with friends or while eating sparingly on the road as He traveled, He never sinned. In fact, nobody ever ate better. Now, that's food for thought.

Some of you may be sitting there thinking, "Wait, what? Surely you don't mean *perfectly*?" Well, in fact, that's exactly what I mean. See, I believe Jesus was perfect in every imaginable way, and that includes how He ate. It's easy to think of Jesus as a healer or speaker, but as a perfect eater? Well, while I know He never ate for vanity or gluttony, the truth is easier to digest when we realize that nothing He ate or didn't eat would prevent Him from reaching the cross for your sins and mine. Sure, I doubt He counted calories, but I do know He led a perfect life, in thought and deed. Knowing that, it's tough to argue that He didn't eat perfectly. After all, Jesus said, "My food is to do the will of Him who sent me and to accomplish His work" (John 4:34).

Now, I admit, I'm leaning on the truth of His perfection pretty heavily to prove a point, but what can His view of food teach us? First and foremost, it should remind us that God looks at the heart, so we might as well get out of the mirror. But it also means that neglecting the body and eating without purpose is a *heart issue*. On one hand, we can't be so focused on our waistline that we fail to see the needs around us, nor can we eat in such a way that we can't function with abundance or fulfill our potential. But isn't it liberating? I believe Jesus enjoyed a good meal with the disciples, and I like to imagine Him leaning back and being the first to doze off after being filled. But humbly, I can also see Him going days *without* food, fasting for Heavenly wisdom for you and for me. And it's when we see food through His eyes that the table clearly comes into focus: food should *fuel* our lives, not *rule* our lives. And that's the purpose of this book you're holding. I want you to embrace food, enjoy food, and command food, learning how it allows you to better serve God and others. My fingers are crossed hoping that you do.

NOW WHAT?

Now what? Have you ever asked yourself that? If so, you're not alone. Not only have I asked myself that question many times, but a few others you might recognize probably have, too. Who comes to mind? Abraham when he reached the altar with Isaac; Moses when he reached the sea; Joshua when they finally reached Jericho. The same question they whispered to themselves after being obedient was the same question the enemy shouted when Jesus was on the cross: *Now what?* In response, God left Heaven's hall for Bethlehem's stall. He then climbed out of his crib and onto the cross. He became the answer to our biggest question and our direst need.

Are you facing a now-what moment? You've finished this

book and you've come to grips with the fact that your health is simultaneously in God's hands and under your care. Because you can't earn Heaven, He's put you in charge of something that requires your *best* effort. And because of that, I've given you mine. You now have in writing the philosophy I apply to my life, the lives of the famous who trust me to help them with their projects, and the tens of thousands of people I speak to on the subject of faith and health. You have my best because I want you to achieve yours.

The PrayFit Diet is the most thorough, the most balanced, the most faith-filled eating plan ever designed. Through it and with it, you can lose as much weight as you desire to lose, in part because you have learned what foods do to the body and for the body. You've learned about the muscle-building and metabolism-boosting properties of protein. Together we've studied the power of carbohydrates and the amazing benefits of healthy fats.

The trinity of protein, fat, and carbs is what God gave us to feast upon. They're His ingredients. He gave earth a kitchen and stocked it full. Upon the cutting board He placed lean cuts of meat. In the garden He planted delicious fruits, vegetables, and herbs. Imagine Him wrapping an apron around His waist, lovingly creating the recipe of our lives. I think one way we can thank Him for our food is to smile as we catch a whiff of it. Don't you?

But friends, the most powerful ingredient He made for us isn't found in the kitchen cupboard. It's not hidden in the fridge or on the top shelf of the pantry. No, the single most important ingredient God provided is *choice*. Choice to choose Him, choice to follow Him, and yes, the choice to honor Him with our bodies, to exercise regularly, and, most important, to eat a balanced life; to see health as a means of praise.

I have said it before, but He's the point of the story. He's the point of this book. And He's the point of our health. The perfect breakdown of macronutrients, the beautifully assembled meal plans and recipes, and the library of knowledge you now have in your hands are exactly what you need for obedience, lower body weight, lower body fat, higher confidence, higher achievement, abundant health, and an extraordinary life. "Now what?" you ask. *Now* you pray and eat with purpose. *Now* you and everything on your table are subject to your faith; a faith that moves mountains and a faith that has moved you to see your body like never before. *Now* you start checking off achieved goals. *Now* you start fending off compliments and giving God the glory for your weight loss. *Now* you start living physically how your soul feels spiritually. Because of your faith, your "Now what?" just became "What's next?" And on that note, I think I'll stop. It's time for dinner. *Thank you, dear Lord, for our food. Amen.*

PrayFit Diet
Frequently Asked Questions

Is Diet Soda Okay for Me to Drink?

If you're comparing diet soda to regular soda, which has roughly 150 calories, then yes. Regular soda is all sugar, all "empty." That said, even though diet sodas don't have all that sugar, they're still jam-packed with the fake, chemically based, artificial stuff. And some diet sodas are packed with things like sodium and even phosphorus, which can limit your body's ability to absorb calcium. So lay off the diet soda, even if it means slowly removing it daily. Try to get down to the point where—at most—you're drinking 1–2 cans a week, if at all.

How many hours a night should I sleep to take advantage of all the great food in the PrayFit diet?

While research varies, one thing we are pretty sure about is that people who lack sleep tend to overeat. There could be plenty of reasons for it, but I tend to believe that if you're tired, you'll make poorer choices and lack willpower. A rested, clear mind is better able to withstand physical obstacles and enjoy triumphs better throughout the day. Some people may need more sleep than others to feel their best, but whatever that number is for you, shoot for it. Let your body have the time it needs to recover, renew, recuperate, and recalibrate.

Is frozen food really that bad for me? Is it okay to occasionally pop things into the microwave?

It depends. (Don't you just love that answer?) Well, here's why. If you're looking for frozen fruits and vegetables, enjoy! Fruits and veggies in the frozen section are just as healthy as the fresh kind, so have at them. And what's great, they'll obviously last longer, and that works well for you when things go in and out of season. All of the same nutrients, vitamins, and minerals in fresh fruit and veggies are available in the frozen section (just be careful with fruit to make sure they're not loaded with artificial sweeteners). Now, before we take a victory lap, avoid the frozen entrees. Those are the ones that are loaded with artificial ingredients and sodium and void of healthy fiber and nutrients.

If one day's meal plan is healthy, why can't I eat the same thing every day if I enjoy it? Won't I lose weight just as easily as long as everything is 33 percent, as you suggest?

I admit, I've been known to find what meals I love and stick with just those. Being a creature of habit, that suits me just fine. However, if you and I stick to the same foods day in and day out, it's likely that we'll miss out on a variety of health-bolstering vitamins and minerals that can only be had through the kind of variety I've outlined in The PrayFit Diet. The constant influx of the vast spectrum of nutritious foods ensures for an adequate helping and will continue to keep your body churning and burning to help you lose or maintain your desired weight. A well-rounded diet is one that teaches you so much about all the food that the good Lord gave us, while providing limitless benefits simultaneously.

Is it important for me to eat before I work out if I do so early in the morning? Or should I just wait and eat after I train? What's best for weight loss?

I've read multiple and conflicting reports about what's best to eat first thing in the morning for optimal weight loss. Some experts say to train on an empty stomach so you'll torch your fat stores. Others say to make sure you take in a fast-digesting protein first thing to help elevate the fat-burning process. My take? I personally prefer to have something in my stomach before I train, regardless of the time of day. If you work out first thing in the morning, be aware that you've just endured an overnight fast, with possibly 7, 8, or 9 hours of food-deprived sleep. Because of that fact, your body is ready for fuel. And if you're about to hit something intense and fun like one of the PrayFit DVDs, your performance may be hindered if you haven't fueled up. My advice is to eat a good, clean protein source, as well as a slow-digesting carbohydrate. You want to have something in your stomach, nothing too heavy to slow you down, but you also don't want to be hungry halfway through your workout. (HINT: Any of our breakfasts will do.)

What about caffeine? Is it safe and will my daily coffee run help me lose weight?
As far as coffee, it's perfectly fine to have a couple cups a day. Coffee is virtually calorie-free and even has antioxidants. But it's more about what you add to your coffee that gets you into trouble. Unless the coffee shop has already loaded your order up with various flavors of sugar and fat, it's more about what you add to the steaming cup of joe that matters most. Bottom line, drink coffee as straight as possible, and do so in moderation. Some people may be pre-exposed to heart conditions that may be worsened with coffee. After all, caffeine is a stimulant.

What if I miss one of the meals on The PrayFit Diet? Have I ruined my day? Can I make up for it at night?
It's true that the meals we've assembled for you will work best if

you spread them out through the day, but if you miss one or two of them, what I don't want you to do is try and make up for it by doubling or tripling your calories in one huge meal at night. If possible, snack on something healthy as soon as you can, which should help curb your hunger before supper, but try to eat a sensible and balanced meal regardless. You can have one of the healthy snacks before bedtime, if you happen to get hungry, but creating an enormous, calorie-rich meal will not help you lose weight and could even hinder that goal. Like putting a massive log on a fire and hoping it burns. No, the better option is to eat a couple of sensible snacks along with one of the perfectly por-tioned PrayFit meals. The next day will be here soon enough.

I'm the only one in my family who needs to lose weight. Should I be the only one enjoying The PrayFit Diet?
Absolutely not. The meals that I've laid out for you in the PrayFit Diet are not only good for you if you're trying to lose weight and gain health, they're ideal for any person who is blessed to sit at your table and eat under your roof. If you have teenagers, their calorie needs may be outside your range, but the PrayFit meals are the same kinds of foods they should be eating. Plainly said, you don't have to create two different dinners! The delicious vari-ety of proteins, fats, and carbs are fit for anyone: husbands, wives, sons, daughters, aunts, and uncles. Because sensible eating is a way of life, there's no reason why those around you should not be eating the PrayFit way, healthy and balanced. Won't it be great to know that everyone you love is honoring the Lord with each meal and living an abundant life?

My work and lifestyle have me eating out a lot. How do I make sure that I'm sticking to what I now know is best for my health?
Going to restaurants doesn't have to wreck your plans. If the healthiest options aren't easy to spot, you can begin with dial-

ing down the portion sizes. Because restaurant plates are bigger than ever and the amount of food so extreme, go ahead and ask for a smaller plate, such as a salad plate. Then don't be shy and transfer food to that plate. Once you realize that you can thrive on less food than restaurants serve, you'll grow more and more accustomed to proper portion sizes. Be thankful that you can ask for a doggy bag without regret or hesitation. And if you remember what I said about counterfeit bills, spotting a fake is about to get easier and easier. The more you study the PrayFit Diet, the easier it will be to be at a restaurant and not only order well, but leave as healthy as you walked in.

I love chocolate, I admit. What is the truth about the "good" chocolate and the "bad" (if there is such a thing)? Can I have it on The PrayFit Diet?
Don't we all love the occasional chocolaty delight? And yes, there is a better chocolate out there. In terms of "better," the darker chocolate devours milk chocolate. The dark stuff has flavonoids that mirror antioxidants and actually help prevent cell damage. Look for chocolate that's high in cacao. The reason it's not as sweet as milk chocolate is it has less sugar and, thus, is a little safer on your overall health. Just be careful not to keep it stored in the pantry—I like to eat it occasionally, as a treat, usually when I'm dining out. Savor it sparingly and enjoy it, but don't have it in the house awaiting your every whim.

I love that my kids are starting to enjoy helping me in the kitchen, but what should they be helping with and what should I save for when they get older?
Indeed, the more time you spend learning and mastering the food in the PrayFit Diet, your enthusiasm will rub off quickly. Kids can have a special time in the kitchen. I remember helping my mom make her classic Chicken Jerusalem dish, and to this day

we compare recipes. But for the little ones, build a kid-friendly kitchen. Make sure all of your measuring cups are plastic and not glass. If your kids are helping you as you cut meat, take the opportunity to talk about food safety; also wash cutting boards and hands thoroughly and often. And I know this next tidbit from experience: make sure your kids understand that just because they don't see a flame on the stove doesn't mean it's not HOT! Take the time to teach them about electric stoves, and always keep processors and blenders unplugged when you're not using them. That one button is just so tempting (so I hear).

Why 33 days? Is there something to that length of time?
Well, first and foremost, I designed it as a thirty-three-day plan to honor the life of Christ. He gave us thirty-three years, and I wanted to glorify that with a thirty-three-day meal plan. But also, as a physiologist, I know that a month-long program has been shown to be a highly effective time frame for people to see change and to create long-lasting habits. So it's both a spiritual and physical number. A number that will forever be etched upon my heart, and hopefully yours, too. It's 33 days for the rest of your God-given, abundant, and glorious life.

Acknowledgments

Michelle Howry, editor supreme—I can't thank you enough for what you've meant to this project. Your amazing heart, leadership, and dedication will be eternally cherished.

The publishing team at Touchstone—Susan Moldow, Stacy Creamer, David Falk, Sally Kim, Jessica Roth, Elaine Wilson, Meredith Vilarello, Cherlynne Li, Ruth Lee-Mui, George Turianski, Mia Crowley-Hald. Without all of you, there is no telling.

Celeste Fine and Sterling Lord Literistic Inc.—you skillfully and gracefully created this partnership. If the words "grateful" and "thankful" have ever fallen short, it's now.

Dana Angelo White—a maestro of recipes. If it calls for a dash of delicious and a pinch of brilliance, there is only one name that can stir it: yours.

Jim Stoppani, PhD—your genius mind has changed many lives, none more than mine. Thank you for laying the groundwork for this book.

Eric Velazquez—what can I say? Good game. This is *me*, pointing at you.

Mom and Dad—dinnertime is still my fondest memory. Your love for the Lord and each other made this book possible. (And don't worry, Mom, your recipes are still safe . . . *with you*.)

And most of all to you, Jesus, my Savior. Thank you for steeping our hearts in grace. May this book help every reader honor you with every meal.

Bibliography

Bosse, John D., and Brian M. Dixon. 2012. "Dietary Protein to Maximize Resistance Training: A Review and Examination of Protein Spread and Change Theories." *Journal of the International Society of Sports Nutrition* 9: 42.

Brattbakk, Hans-Richard, et al. 2013. "Balanced Caloric Macronutrient Composition Downregulates Immunological Gene Expression in Human Blood Cells—Adipose Tissue Diverges." OMICS 17 (1): 41–52.

Evans, Ellen M., et al. 2012. "Effects of Protein Intake and Gender on Body Composition Changes: A Randomized Clinical Weight Loss Trial." *Nutrition & Metabolism* 9: 55.

Layman, Donald K., et al. 2003. "A Reduced Ratio of Dietary Carbohydrate to Protein Improves Body Composition and Blood Lipid Profiles During Weight Loss in Adult Women." *Journal of Nutrition* 133 (2): 411–17.

Lowery, Lonnie M., and Devia Lorena. 2009. "Dietary Protein Safety and Resistance Exercise: What Do We Really Know?" *Journal of the International Society of Sports Nutrition* 6: 3.

Mahon, Anne K., et al. 2007. "Protein Intake During Energy Restriction: Effects on Body Composition and Markers of Metabolic and Cardiovascular Health in Postmenopausal Women." *Journal of the American College of Nutrition* 26 (2): 182–89.

Mojtahedi, Mina C., et al. 2011. "The Effects of a Higher Protein Intake During Energy Restriction on Changes in Body Composition and Physical Function in Older Women." *Journals of Gerontology, Series A: Biological Sciences and Medical Sciences* 66A (11): 1218–25.

"Study: Obesity Adds $190 Billion in Health Costs." http://www.nbcnews.com/id/47211549/ns/health-diet_and_nutrition/t/study-obesity-adds-billion-health-costs/#.Un3c5RyeGnw.

Volek, J. S., et al. 2004. "Comparison of Energy-Restricted Very Low-Carbohydrate and Low-Fat Diets on Weight Loss and Body Composition in Overweight Men and Women." *Nutrition & Metabolism* 1: 13.

Index

Page numbers in *italics* indicate recipe locations

About the Authors

JIMMY PEÑA is a *New York Times* bestselling author, the founder of PrayFit (www.prayfit.com), and has been the exercise physiologist to Tyler Perry, Mario Lopez, and LL Cool J. He earned his bachelor's degree in business management from Baylor University in 1994 and his master's degree in clinical exercise physiology from the University of Texas at Tyler in 1998.

Jimmy coauthored the *New York Times* bestseller *Extra Lean* by Mario Lopez, and he designed the women's training programs for LL Cool J's *New York Times* bestseller *Platinum Workout*. Jimmy is also the author of the Amazon bestseller *PrayFit: Your Guide to a Healthy Body and a Stronger Faith in 28 Days* (Regal Books).

Mentioned by Tyler Perry on *The Tonight Show* with Jay Leno, ABC's *The View*, and CNN's *Piers Morgan*, and seen on HBO's Pay-Per-View Championship Boxing, Prayfit's popularity paved the way for two workout DVDs with Lionsgate Entertainment, the first of which (*PrayFit: 33-Day Total Body Challenge*) was released in December 2011 and remained Amazon's #1 Hottest New Release in Faith for fifty-three days. The second DVD, released December 2012, hit #1 on Amazon in January 2013, and has remained one of Amazon's bestselling DVDs since.

Jimmy was recently named the first advisory board member of Pastor Rick Warren's The Daniel Plan weight-loss initiative. Jimmy Peña is rapidly becoming a keynote speaker of choice in venues ranging from churches, businesses, expos, and conferences. His storytelling approach, along with his targeted and motivational message of faith and health, is nothing short of captivating.

ERIC VELAZQUEZ, NSCA-CPT, is a veteran health and fitness writer and has worked for several of the industry's top fitness publications, including *Muscle and Fitness, FLEX,* and *MuscleMag.* In 2005, while at *Muscle and Fitness,* he met Jimmy and was recruited to help lay the foundation for PrayFit. Now charged with crafting PrayFit's message editorially, Eric has also worked as a writer for numerous other sports and fitness titles, including *Life Extension, Defense Media Network, Swimming World, Muscle and Performance, PowerBar, Everlast Magazine, Water Polo Around the Globe,* and *Angels Magazine.* He has produced fitness content for a wide spectrum of audiences, from the hard-core followers of elite bodybuilding to thirtysomething weekend warriors just looking to get an edge.

DANA ANGELO WHITE, MS, RD, ATC, is a registered dietitian, certified athletic trainer, and nutrition and fitness consultant for international food companies, restaurants, and marketing firms. She specializes in culinary nutrition, recipe development, and sports nutrition. Dana works closely with chefs and authors to develop creative and healthy recipes for cookbooks, marketing campaigns, and restaurant menus. She is currently the nutrition expert for FoodNetwork.com and has worked as media spokesperson for *Cooking Light* magazine. She has appeared on *Good Day Street Talk,* FoodNetwork.com, *Access Hollywood,* and *GMA Health,* and is the president of Dana White Nutrition, Inc. Her recipes and articles have been featured on FoodNetwork.com, CookingLight.com, DietTV.com, and VarsityParenting.com, and in *Today's Dietitian, Shape, Seventeen, Prevention,* and *Maxim.* She created meal plans and recipes for books including *Energy to Burn: The Ultimate Food and Nutrition Guide to Fuel Your Active Life* and *Extra Lean* by Mario Lopez. She also worked with Harvard Medical School's Center for Health and the Global Environment to create the Healthy Harvest Food Guides, to educate consumers how to purchase and prepare seasonal foods. Dana earned her master's degree in nutrition education from Teachers' College–Columbia University and her bachelor's degree in sports medicine from Quinnipiac University, where she currently works as the sports RD for Division 1 athletes and as an assistant clinical faculty member in the sports medicine program and school of medicine. She resides in Fairfield, Connecticut, with her husband, two daughters, and Boston terrier, Violet Pickles. For more information, visit her official website at www.danawhitenutrition.com.

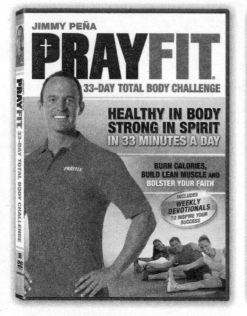
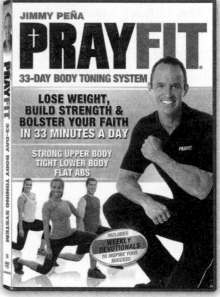
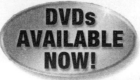